MEN

11.00 a

IN FOCUS

Titles published in the series:

* Antigen-presenting Cells
* Complement 2nd edn
Cytokines and Cytokine Receptors
DNA Replication
DNA Structure and Recognition
DNA Topology
Enzyme Kinetics
Gene Structure and Transcription 2nd edn
Genetic Engineering
Growth Factors
* Immune Recognition
Intracellular Protein Degradation
* B Lymphocytes
* Lymphokines
Membrane Structure and Function
Molecular Basis of Inherited Disease 2nd edn
Molecular Genetic Ecology
Protein Biosynthesis
Protein Engineering
Protein Structure
Protein Targeting and Secretion
Regulation of Enzyme Activity
* The Thymus

* Published in association with the British Society for Immunology.

Series editors

David Rickwood

Department of Biology, University of Essex, Wivenhoe Park, Colchester, Essex CO4 3SQ, UK

David Male

Institute of Psychiatry, De Crespigny Park, Denmark Hill, London SE5 8AF, UK

COMPLEMENT
Second edition

S. K. A. Law and K. B. M. Reid

MRC Immunochemistry Unit, Department of Biochemistry,
University of Oxford, South Parks Road, Oxford OX1 3QU, UK

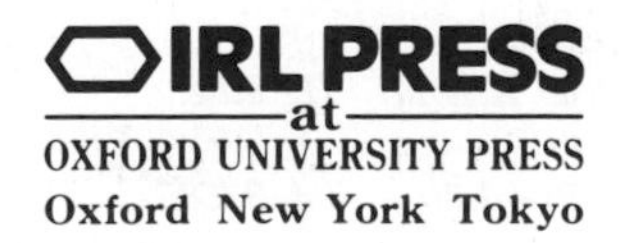

Oxford University Press, Walton Street, Oxford OX2 6DP

Oxford New York
Athens Auckland Bangkok Bombay
Calcutta Cape Town Dar es Salaam Delhi
Florence Hong Kong Istanbul Karachi
Kuala Lumpur Madras Madrid Melbourne
Mexico City Nairobi Paris Singapore
Taipei Tokyo Toronto
and associated companies in
Berlin Ibadan

Oxford is a trade mark of Oxford University Press

In Focus is a registered trade mark of the Chancellor, Masters, and Scholars of the University of Oxford trading as Oxford University Press

Published in the United States
by Oxford University Press Inc., New York

First edition published 1988 by IRL Press Ltd
Second edition published 1995

A catalogue record for this book is available from the British Library

Library of Congress Cataloging in Publication Data
Law, S.K.A.
Complement / S.K.A. Law and K.B.M. Reid—2nd ed.
p. cm.—(In focus)
Includes bibliographical references and index.
1. Complement (Immunology) I. Reid, K.B.M. II. Title.
III. Series: In focus (Oxford, England)
QR185.8.C6L38 1995 616.079—dc20 94-37685
ISBN 0 19 963356 8

Typeset by Footnote Graphics, Warminster, Wiltshire
Printed in Malta by Interprint

Preface to the second edition

Complement is a group of proteins that form the principal effector arm of the humoral immune system. It was initially recognized, at the end of the last century, as the heat-labile factor in serum required along with heat-stable antibody, for bactericidal activity. Today, more than 30 proteins, both in serum and on the cell surface, have been shown to be closely involved with the complement system. By a series of specific activation steps, which are triggered by the presence of foreign entities, via either the classical, the alternative, or the lectin pathway, the complement proteins mediate a set of activities ranging from the initiation of inflammation, neutralization of pathogens, clearance of immune complexes, disruption of cell membranes, and regulation of the immune response.

The use of recombinant DNA techniques has allowed the rapid determination of the primary structures of nearly all the known complement components, control proteins, and receptors associated with the system, as well as their gene structures and chromosome locations within the human genome. Each complement protein/receptor can now be assigned to a distinct superfamily of structurally related molecules and this provides some insight into the structure/function relationships and the evolutionary aspects of the system. The ability to produce relatively large amounts of complement proteins, their fragments, and variant forms by expressing them in bacterial, or eukaryotic, systems has already allowed the three-dimensional structure determination of several components or fragments and the assignment of active determinants in these proteins. The current interest clearly lies in the assessment of some of the possible clinical therapeutic uses of these expressed products. In this book we present a brief introduction to the complement system, covering the basic biochemistry and activation pathways, and discuss the different families of proteins in the system and how they interact with each other to mediate the various functions in host defence.

S.K.A. Law
K.B.M. Reid

Acknowledgements

We thank Margery Reid for typing an initial draft of the revised version and Alison Marsland for organizing the reference list.

Contents

Abbreviations

C	complement component
C1-Inh	C1-inhibitor
C3NeF	C3 nephritic factor
C4bp	C4 binding protein
CCP	complement control protein
CR	complement receptor
CVF	cobra venom factor
DAF	decay accelerating factor
EBV	Epstein–Barr virus
EDTA	ethylenediaminetetraacetate
EGF	epidermal growth factor
FcR	Fc receptor
GPI	glycosyl phosphatidylinositol
HANE	hereditary angioneurotic oedema
HIV	human immunodeficiency virus
Ig	immunoglobulin
IL	interleukin
LDLr	low density lipoprotein receptor
LFA-1	leukocyte function associated antigen 1
LHR	long homologous repeat
α_2M	α_2-macroglobulin
MAC	membrane attack complex
MASP	MBP-associated serine protease
MBP	mannan binding protein
MCP	membrane cofactor protein
MHC	major histocompatibility complex
NMR	nuclear magnetic resonance
P	properdin
PNH	paroxysmal nocturnal haemoglobinuria
RCA	regulators of complement activation
SCr	scavenger receptor
SLE	systemic lupus erythematosus
TAPA-1	target for antiproliferative antibody antigen-1
TNF	tumour necrosis factor

TSR	thrombospondin repeat
VWF	von Willebrand factor

Single-letter codes of the amino acids

A	Alanine	C	Cysteine	D	Aspartic acid	E	Glutamic acid
F	Phenylalanine	G	Glycine	H	Histidine	I	Isoleucine
K	Lysine	L	Leucine	M	Methionine	N	Asparagine
P	Proline	Q	Glutamine	R	Arginine	S	Serine
T	Threonine	V	Valine	W	Tryptophan	Y	Tyrosine

1

Complement

1. Introduction

Complement is a major defence and clearance system in the bloodstream which can be activated via immunoglobulins once a foreign particle or organism has been recognized by antibody. Direct activation of the system can also take place if the particle provides a suitable site for the amplified self-activation of the early acting components. Complement was first described in the 1890s as being principally a heat-labile bactericidal activity in serum which was triggered after the heat-stable antibodies had recognized and bound to the invading microorganisms. By the 1920s evidence was available showing that this heat-labile bactericidal activity required the presence of at least four serum fractions but, due to the lack of rigorous protein purification methods, little advance was made in the chemical characterization of the numerous components of the system until the early 1960s. Once techniques such as ion-exchange chromatography were readily available it became clear [mainly as a result of the work carried out in the laboratories of R.A.Nelson (1) and H.J. Müller-Eberhard (2)] that the immunologically triggered pathway of complement activation (the classical pathway) is composed of eleven distinct plasma proteins (3). A second activation pathway (the alternative pathway), not necessarily involving antibody, had been proposed by Pillemer in the late 1950s (4, 5), but it was not until almost 1970 that evidence of the existence of this pathway was finally accepted (6). Detailed structural, functional and biosynthetic studies on the various components and control proteins regulating the pathways were carried out in the 1970s. This paved the way for the molecular cloning at the cDNA level of all the components, control proteins, and most of the receptors associated with the pathways, several of which have only recently been fully described. Also, the recent demonstration of an antibody-independent route of activation of the classical pathway, via a serum lectin and a newly described serum protease, is an example of one of several important findings which has emerged since the first edition of this book. This new activation route could provide rapid defence against pathogens via innate immune mechanisms, rather than being dependent upon the generation of specific antibodies. Thus, in view of the significant amount of new information regarding the structure, function, biosynthesis, and genetics which has recently been generated about complement components and receptors, it seems appropriate to update this short but hopefully comprehensive general introduction to the system.

1.1 Nomenclature

All proteins associated with the complement system are listed in *Tables 1.1–1.3*. The plasma proteins of the classical pathway and terminal attack complex are defined as 'components' and each is given a number and prefixed by 'C'. Thus, C1–C9 are the components of the classical pathway and terminal membrane attack complex. The membrane attack complex (MAC) is composed of activated C5 along with components C6–C9. All these components are distinct plasma glycoproteins with the exception of C1, which is a complex of three glycoproteins, the subcomponents of C1: C1q, C1r, and C1s. Where there is more than one polypeptide chain within an unactivated component they are designated α, β, and γ, an exception is the C1q molecule for which the designation A, B, and C has been given for the three types of polypeptide chains found in the molecule. Two of the proteins of the alternative pathway are designated as 'factors' and each is given a letter: factor B and factor D. A third protein of the alternative pathway is properdin. Acceptable abbreviations for these alternative pathway proteins are B, D, and P. Two of the control proteins are also designated as 'factors': factor I and factor H, while the other control proteins are usually referred to by abbreviations of their trivial names, for example C1-Inh for C1-inhibitor.

There are seven enzymes, of the serine protease type, associated with the activation and control of the pathways (*Tables 1.1* and *1.2*). Activation steps involving these enzymes are always achieved by very specific limited proteolysis, with only one bond being split at any one step. Control of the activated components is also achieved by splitting of only a limited number of bonds. The enzymatically active forms of components generally have a bar over the symbol, for example $C\overline{1r}$, $C\overline{1s}$. A complex containing an active site may also be written with a bar over the whole complex, for example $C\overline{1}$ and $C\overline{3bBb}$. Fragments generated by limited proteolysis are indicated by suffixed lower case letters, for example C4a and C4b for the activation fragments of C4. The receptors are usually given as abbreviations of their trivial names, for example complement receptor type 1, the C4b/C3b receptor, is given as CR1.

It should be noted that C4 is activated prior to C2 and C3 and this is merely a reflection of the original numbering given to the fractions containing these components before the order of activation was clearly identified.

1.2 General outline of the complement system

Complement can be activated by two distinct routes, the classical and alternative pathways (*Figure 1.1*). The component C3 is a major plasma glycoprotein

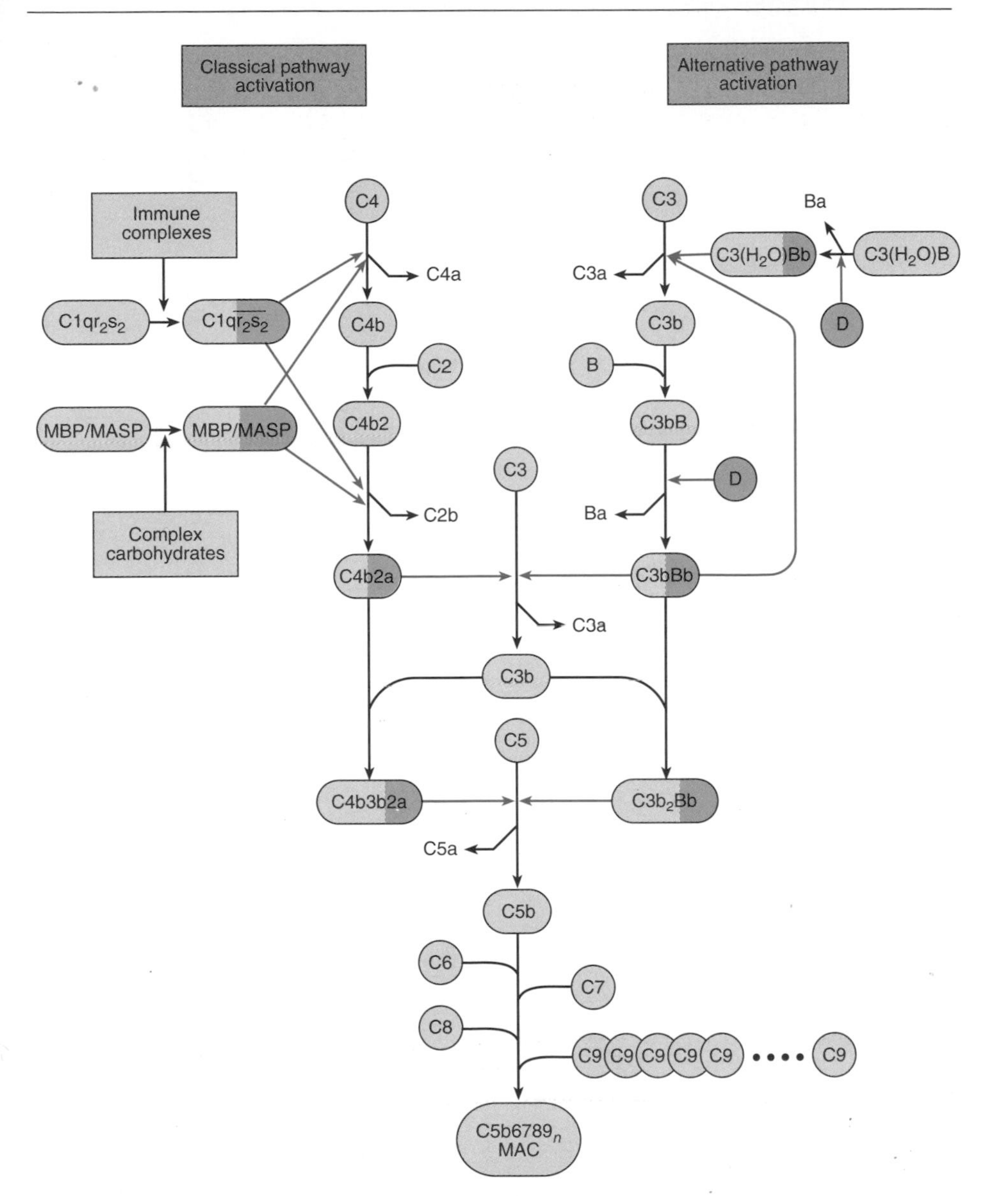

Figure 1.1. The activation steps of the classical pathway (left) are triggered by immune complexes or by complex carbohydrates via the lectin pathway, while the alternative pathway (right) is activated by a wide variety of compounds and cell surfaces. The number of C9 molecules (*n*) within the $C5b6789_n$ complex can vary between 1 and 18. Enzymatic cleavage is indicated as solid orange lines, and the enzymatically active components are shaded orange.

Table 1.1 Plasma proteins involved in the activation of the complement system

	M_r (kDa)	Number of chains in plasma form prior to activation	M_r of individual chains (kDa)	Chromosome location of gene	Plasma concentation		Enzymatic site in activated form (+) (and natural substrate split)
					μg ml^{-1}	μM	
Classical pathway							
C1q	462	18 (6 A + 6 B + 6 C)	A: 26.5	1p34.1–36.3	80	0.17	–
			B: 26.5	1p34.1–36.3			
			C: 24	1p34.1–36.3			
C1r[a]	83	1		12p13	50	0.30	+ (C1r, C1s)
C1s[a]	83	1		12p13	50	0.30	+ (C4, C2)
C4	205	3 (β + α + γ)[b]	α: 97	6p21.3	600	3.00	–
			β: 75				
			γ: 33				
C2	102	1		6p21.3	20	0.20	+ (C3, C5)
C3	185	2 (β + α)[b]	α: 110	19	1300	7.02	–
			β: 75				
Lectin route							
MBP[c]	540	18	32	10	1[e]	0.002	–
MASP[d]	94	1		n.k.	n.k.		+ (C4, C2)

Alternative pathway							
Factor D	24	1		n.k.	1	0.04	+ (B)
Factor B	92	1		6p21.3	210	2.20	+ (C3, C5)
C3	185	2 (β + α)[b]		19	1300	7.02	–
Terminal components							
C5	190	2 (β + α)[b]	α: 115 β: 75	9q 32–34	70	0.37	–
C6	120	1		5q	64	0.53	–
C7	110	1		5q	56	0.51	+
C8	150	3 (α + β + γ)	α: 64 β: 64 γ: 22	1p34 1p34 9q	55	0.36	–
C9	71	1		5p13	59	0.83	–

n.k. = not known.

[a] C1r and C1s are present in plasma either as a complex with C1q in the composition C1q–$C1r_2$–$C1s_2$ or in the absence of C1q as a C1s–C1r–C1r–C1s tetramer (see text and *Figure 2.2*).

[b] These chains are initially synthesized as a single chain precursor molecule in the order shown.

[c] MBP = Mannan binding protein.

[d] MASP = MBP-associated serine protease.

[e] The plasma concentration of MBP varies widely in different individuals over the range of 0.1–5.0 $\mu g\ ml^{-1}$ i.e. 0.002–0.01 μM

Table 1.2 Plasma proteins involved in control of the complement system

Protein	M_r (kDa)	Approximate plasma concentration		Specficity	Chromosome location of gene	Role
		μg ml^{-1}	μM			
C1-Inh	110	200	1.82	C1r, C1s	11p11.2–13	Forms covalent 1:1 complex with both C1r and C1s and removes them from complex
C4 binding protein (C4bp)[a]	500	250	0.45	C4b	1q32	Accelerates decay from C4b2a and acts as cofactor in the cleavage of C4b by factor I
Factor H	150	480	3.20	C3b	1q	Accelerates decay of C3bBb and acts as cofactor in the cleavage of C3b by factor I
Factor I	88	35	0.39	C4b, C3b	4q24–26	Protease which inactivates C4b and C3b with the aid of cofactors C4bp, H, CR1 and MCP[b]
Properdin[c]	220	10	0.05	C3bBb	Xp11.23–11.3	Positive regulator of the alternative pathway which stabilizes the C3/C5 convertases.
Anaphylatoxin inactivator[d]	310	35	0.11	C3a, C4a, C5a	n.k.	Carboxypeptidase which inactivates the anaphylatoxins C3a, C4a, and C5a by removal of a C-terminal arginine residue in each
S-protein (vitronectin)	83	505	6.08	C5b-7	17q11	Up to three molecules of S-protein bind to C5b-7 preventing the complex from binding to cell surfaces
SP40,40	80	50	1.20	C5b6	8p21	Acts after the fluid-phase assembly of C5b6 and prevents the hydrophilic– amphiphatic transition which C5b-7 undergoes prior to membrane insertion

n.k. = not known.

[a] C4 binding protein is disulphide-bonded heptamer of identical α subunits each of ~70 kDa, or one of the α subunits is replaced by a β subunit of 45 kDa to form a 6α1β complex. The gene of the β subunit is located to within 10 kb of the α subunit genre

[b] MCP = membrane cofactor protein

is a multimer of a 45 kDa subunit: the predominant form contains three or four subunits.

oxin inactivator contains three different polypeptides of M_r 83, 55, and 49 kDa. The stoichiometric composition of these polypeptides in the not clear.

Table 1.3 Membrane-associated molecules which act as receptors/regulators for fragments[a] of activated complement components

Membrane molecule		*Mr*[b] (kDa)	Fragment specificity	Chromosome location of gene	Principal roles	Major human cell types positive
Complement receptor type 1 (CR1) (four structural allotypes)	type D type B type A type C	250 220 190 160	C3b, C4b	1q32	Regulation of C3b breakdown, binding of immune complexes to erythrocytes, phagocytosis, and accelerates decay of C3/C5 convertases	E, B, G, M
Complement receptor type 2 (CR2)		145	C3d, C3dg, iC3b	1q32	Regulation of B cell functions, Epstein–Barr virus receptor	B
Membrane cofactor protein (MCP)		45–70	C3b, C4b	1q32	Regulation of C3b breakdown	B, T, N, M
Decay accelerating factor (DAF)		70	C4b2a, C3bBb	1q32	Accelerates decay of C3/C5-convertases	E, L, P
Complement receptor type 3 (CR3)	(α) (β)	165 95	iC3b	16p11–13.1 21q22.3	Phagocytosis	G, M, ϕ
Glycoprotein p150,95	(α) (β)	150 95	iC3b	16p11–13.1 21q22.3	Monocyte migration	G, M, ϕ
C3a/C4a receptor		n.k.	C3a, C4a	n.k.	Binding of anaphylatoxins C3a and C4a	G, A, P
C5a receptor		~45	C5a, C5a-des arg	n.k.	Binding of anaphylatoxin C5a	G, A, M, ϕ, P
C1q receptor		~65	C1q (collagen region)	n.k.	Mediates binding of immune complexes to phagocytic cells. Inhibition of interleukin-1 expression by B lymphocytes	B, M, ϕ, P, D
Homologous restriction factor		65	C8, C9	n.k.	Prevention of formation of MAC on homologous cells	E
CD59		20	C5b-8	11p13	Prevention of formation of MAC on homologous cells	E, R, and most other cell types

n.k. = not known.
Human cell types: E, erythrocytes; B, B lymphocytes; T, T lymphocytes; M, monocytes; ϕ, macrophages; G, granulocytes; N, neutrophils; L, leukocytes; P, platelets; A, mast cells; D, endothelial cells; R, renal cells.
[a] Receptors for intact factor H and Ba have been found on monocytes, B lymphocytes, and neutrophils.
[b] All appear to be single chain molecules except CR3 and p150,95 which have non-covalently linked α and β subunits.

(present at a concentration of 1.3 mg ml^{-1}) and it plays a central role in the system, being common to both pathways. C3, along with the other 14 plasma glycoproteins, including MBP (mannan binding protein) and MASP (MBP-associated serine protease), shown in *Figure 1.1* and *Table 1.1*, constitute the 15 components of the pathways. It should be noted that the three chains of C1q, A, B, and C, and the three subunits of C8, α, β, and γ, are all distinct gene products. Components C5–C9 are designated the terminal components which form the MAC (membrane attack complex), which is common to both pathways and which is responsible for target cell damage and lysis. Other biologically important functions mediated by the complement system include (i) the low molecular weight (M_r~9000 Da) anaphylatoxins C3a, C4a, and C5a, which promote smooth muscle contraction and increase vascular permeability; (ii) the large C4b and C3b fragments, which are involved in binding to the complement activator and can thereafter interact with specific receptors to allow efficient clearance of the activating cell or particle including viruses; and (iii) degradation fragments of C3b (iC3b, C3dg, C3d), which are also important in the clearance of immune aggregates and the triggering of receptor mediated activities including the regulation of the immune response.

Control of the activated components is mediated partly via the seven control proteins present in plasma (*Table 1.2*) and partly by a variety of membrane bound control proteins and receptors (*Table 1.3*). Since many of the activation and control steps involve specific limited proteolysis, it is useful to identify clearly which of the components and control proteins are enzymes. Activation of pro-enzymes C1r, C1s (of the C1 complex), MASP (of the MBP–MASP complex), and C2 leads to the formation of enzyme complexes which split C3 and C5. Factors B and D of the alternative pathway are also synthesized as pro-enzymes, although factor D appears to circulate in the blood primarily in its activated form. When factor B is complexed to C3b or C3(H_2O) (see Chapter 2, Section 3), it can be split and activated by factor D to yield eventually the enzyme complexes of the alternative pathway which act on C3 and C5 in an analogous manner to those generated by the classical pathway. After splitting of C5 no other proteolytic events are considered to take place and the lytic C5b-9 complex (MAC) is generated by a self-assembly mechanism.

2. Further reading

Kinoshita,T. (1991). *Immunol. Today*, **12,** No 9 (Entire issue).
Müller-Eberhard,H.J. (1988). *Annu. Rev. Biochem.*, **57,** 321.
Müller-Eberhard,H.J. and Meischer,P.A. (eds) (1985). *Complement.* Springer, Berlin.
Reid,K.B.M. and Porter,R.R. (1981). *Annu. Rev. Biochem.*, **50,** 433.
Ross,G.D. (ed.) (1986). *Immunobiology of the complement system: an introduction for research and clinical medicine.* Academic Press, New York.
Whaley,K. (ed.) (1987). *Complement in health and disease.* MTP, Lancaster.
Whaley,K., Loos,M., and Weiler,J.M. (eds) (1993). *Complement in health and disease.* Immunology and Medicine Series Vol. 20, Kluwer Academic, London.

2.1 Methods

Harrison,R.A. and Lachmann,P.J. (1986). In *Handbook of experimental immunology* (ed. D.M.Weir, L.A.Herzenberg, C.Blackwell, and L.A.Herzenberg), p. 39.1. Blackwell Scientific Publications, Oxford.

Whaley,K. (ed.) (1985). *Methods in complement for clinical immunologists*. Churchill Livingstone Longman Group, Edinburgh.

3. References

1. Nelson,D.S. (1964). *Adv. Immunol.*, **3,** 131.
2. Müller-Eberhard,H.J. (1965). *Adv. Immunol.*, **8,** 1.
3. Nelson,R.A. Jr., Jensen,J., Gigli,I., and Tamura,N. (1966). *Immunochemistry*, **3,** 111.
4. Pillemer,L., Blum,L., Lepow,I.H., Ross,O.A., Todd,E.W., and Wardlaw,A.C. (1954). *Science*, **120,** 279.
5. Pillemer,L. (1955). *Trans. N.Y. Acad. Sci.*, **17,** 526.
6. Lepow,I.H. (1980). *J. Immunol.*, **125,** 471.

2

Activation and control of the complement system

1. Activation of the classical pathway

The classical pathway is considered to be activated *in vivo* primarily by the interaction of the C1q portion of the C1 complex with immune complexes or aggregates containing IgG or IgM. Activation of C1 can also be achieved by its direct interaction with a variety of polyanions (such as bacterial lipopolysaccharides, DNA, and RNA), certain small polysaccharides, viral membranes, C-reactive protein, etc., but the physiological importance of this type of activation is not clear. The C1q molecule, which contains no enzymatic activity, is the portion of the C1 complex which is involved in the recognition and binding of immunoglobulin activators (1) and also a wide variety of non-immune activators (2). The C1q molecule has an unusual shape, being composed of six globular 'heads' each connected by strands to a central fibril-like region, (*Figure 2.1*, see

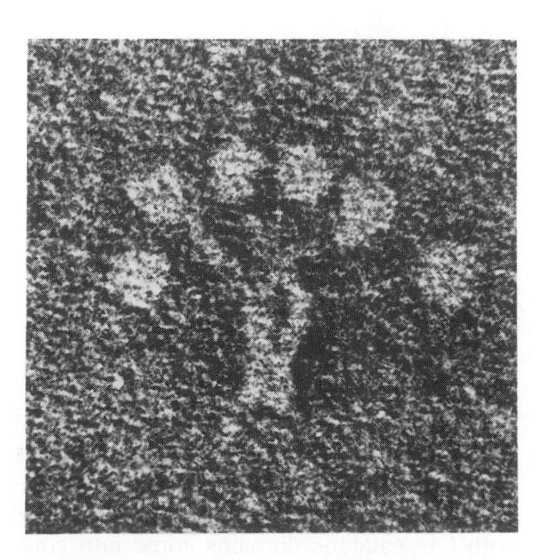

Figure 2.1. Electron micrograph of a C1q molecule showing the six globular 'heads' and the fibril-like collagen region. (From ref. 52, with permission.)

also Chapter 3, Section 1), composed of collagen-like triple helical structures. The enzymatic activity of C1 is derived by activation of the two molecules of pro-enzyme C1r and two molecules of pro-enzyme C1s in the $C1r_2$–$C1s_2$ Ca^{2+}-dependent complex. The purified $C1r_2$–$C1s_2$ complex has an almost rod-like, elongated shape when viewed in the electron microscope, both C1r and C1s being composed of two globular domains connected by an elongated structure (*Figure 2.2*), the larger of the globular domains being considered to contain the catalytic site in activated C1r or C1s. A model for the C1 complex, in which the $C1r_2$–$C1s_2$ complex adopts a distorted 'figure-of-eight' structure with the smaller 'interaction' domains located outside the C1q collagen-like strands while the catalytic domains remain closely associated within the collagen-like cage, is shown in *Figure 2.2*.

Activation of the C1 complex is under the control of the C1-inhibitor (C1-Inh) (3) which binds covalently with the activated C1r and C1s and rapidly removes them from the antibody–antigen–C1q complex. The inhibitory effect of C1-Inh can be overcome by efficient activators of the classical pathway such as immune complexes. The 'heads' of C1q show a weak binding to the Fc region of mono-

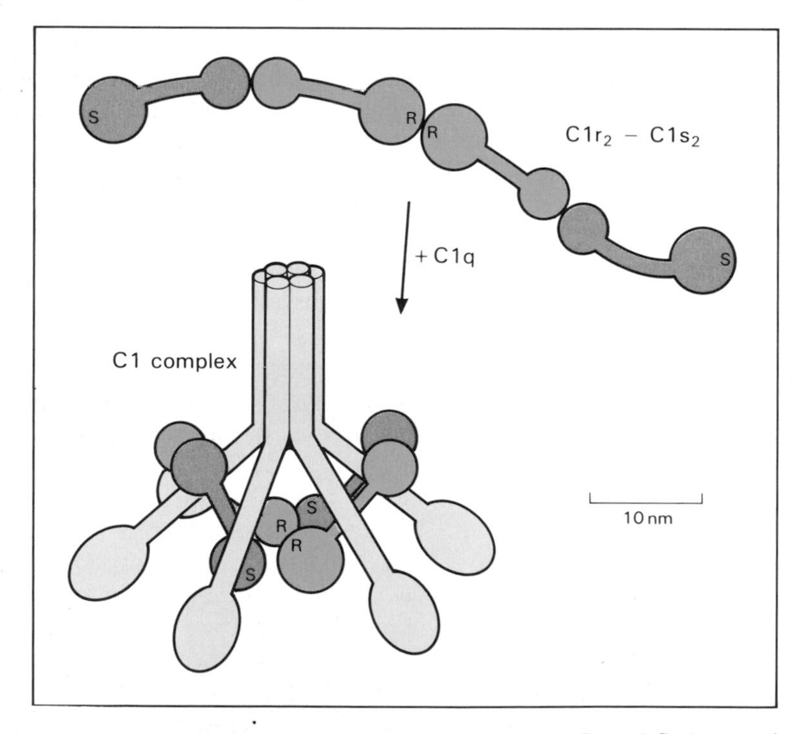

Figure 2.2. Model of $C1r_2$–$C1s_2$ and the C1 complex. R and S denote the larger catalytic domains of C1r and C1s. It is postulated that the C1 complex is formed by placing the rod-like $C1r_2$–$C1s_2$ across the arms of C1q and bending back around two opposite arms so that both C1s catalytic domains come into contact with the centrally located catalytic domains of C1r (adapted from ref. 53).

meric IgG whereas on the presentation of multiple Fc sites, present on aggregated IgG in the immune complexes, the strength of the binding of the C1q 'heads' to the multiple Fc regions is dramatically increased. Different IgG isotypes vary in their ability to bind to C1q and activate complement. In man, IgG1 and IgG3 are active, IgG2 is less active, and IgG4 inactive. In the case of IgM it is apparently the exposure of binding sites in the Fc regions on interaction with large antigens which allows tight IgM–C1q binding to take place. Thus on the interaction of probably two or more of the 'heads' of C1q with a suitable activator, a conformational change may be induced within the C1 complex releasing it from the inhibitory effect of C1-Inh and allowing auto-activation of pro-enzyme C1r to take place. This is rapidly followed by the activation of pro-enzyme C1s by the C$\overline{1r}$ due to the close association of the active site of C$\overline{1r}$ and the activation site of C1s within the collagen-like 'arms' of C1q (*Figure 2.2*).

The three-chain C4 molecule is then split by C$\overline{1s}$ at a single point in its α chain to yield the C4a anaphylatoxin (M_r 9000 Da) and the large C4b fragment. The C4b molecule does not contain an enzymatic site but fulfils at least three important binding functions: (i) freshly activated C4b has the capacity to bind covalently to hydroxyl or amino groups through a reactive acyl group in its α′ chain (see Section 2); (ii) bound C4b can interact with the CR1 receptor (see Section 6.3) found on a variety of phagocytic cells and could play an important role in immune clearance; and (iii) C4b can also interact with the N-terminal C2b domain of pro-enzyme C2 in an Mg^{2+}-dependent fashion. If the binding of C2 to C4b occurs close to the activated C1s then C2 is split at one point to yield the non-catalytic C2b (M_r 30 000 Da) and the C-terminal catalytic C2a (M_r 70 000 Da). The C2b chain is not required for the C3 convertase activity which is mediated via the catalytic site in C2a in the C$\overline{4b2a}$ complex.

Activation of the C1 complex can also be initiated by direct interaction with a variety of non-immune activators such as C-reactive protein, DNA, amyloid P component, and bacterial endotoxins. These molecules all appear to bind to the collagen-like regions of C1q and cause activation of the $C1r_2$–$C1s_2$ complex to take place in a similar fashion to that seen on interaction of the globular heads of C1q, in the C1 complex, with immune aggregates. The physiological importance of this type of non-immune activation of the classical pathway is not entirely clear but, for example, levels of C-reactive protein are markedly raised during inflammation and therefore its involvement in complement activation leading to complement-dependent opsonization and clearance of potentially lethal *pneumococcal* infections (4) indicates that this is an important route in antibody-independent, complement-mediated host defence. Recently another antibody-dependent route of activation of complement has been described which bypasses the use of the C1 complex and makes use of a serum lectin (mannan binding protein or MBP) and a newly described serum protease (MBP-associated serine protease, or MASP, originally described as the M_r 100 000 Da component of Ra-reactive factor) (5). The MBP–MASP complex can activate C4 and C2 (see *Figure 1.1*) once the MBP has bound to suitable carbohydrate ligands present, for example, on the cell surfaces of bacteria or viruses. In addition to possessing carbohydrate binding modules, the MBP molecule contains triple-helical collagen-like regions and thus has an overall structural similarity to C1q. The MASP enzyme is similar in its overall structure to C1r and C1s and therefore there are very clear structural as well as functional similarities between C1q–$C1r_2$–$C1s_2$ and MBP–MASP complexes. In view of the similarity between MASP and C1r and C1s it is perhaps not surprising that it has been reported that MBP can also interact with $C1r_2$–$C1s_2$ and bring about activation of C1s (6). The MBP molecule can interact with the C1q receptor and thus in addition to being involved in complement activation it can present the target, which contains the carbohydrate ligand, to cells carrying the C1q receptor. The serum levels of MBP are approximately 80-fold lower than those of C1q (see *Table 1.1*), but, until the relative efficiencies of the MBP–MASP and C1 complexes, in the activation of C4, and their relative susceptibilities to inhibition by serum inhibitors (such as C1-Inh), are known it is difficult to assess the physiological importance of the MPB–MASP complex. However, an antibody-independent pathway which has the potential to provide rapid complement-mediated defence in the blood may well be important in immunodeficient individuals and the very young who have not yet developed a mature immune system (7).

2. Central role of C3

C3 holds a key position in the complement system since the classical and the alternative pathways merge at the C3 activation step. In the classical pathway, the C3-convertase is the enzyme complex $C\overline{4b2a}$ which activates C3 by the proteolytic cleavage of C3 into C3a and C3b (8). C3a is an anaphylatoxin that consists of the first 77 amino acids of the α chain of C3; the remainder of the molecule is C3b. The removal of C3a induces a conformational change in the C3b portion of the molecule which leads to the exposure of an internal thiolester (9), which is buried and quite inaccessible in native C3 (10). The exposed thiolester is extremely reactive with nucleophiles, including water and molecules bearing hydroxyl or amino groups. If these molecules are found on the cell surface, C3b will become covalently bound to the cell by an ester or an amide bond (*Figure 2.3*) (11, 12).

Thus, the internal thiolester confers C3, upon its activation, with the potential to form covalently linked complexes with any nucleophile, including the hydroxyl and amino groups on any biological surfaces of foreign or host origin. Although its versatility to bind to all types of foreign cells is desirable, its binding to host cells must be minimized. The safeguard, however, is intrinsic to the thiolester itself. Once activated, the thiolester is extremely reactive. Water, at a concentration of 55 M in the medium, readily hydrolyses the thiolester and effectively puts a limit on the spatial range of the activated C3b. C3b activated at the surface of a foreign cell, via either the classical or the alternative pathway of complement, is largely restricted to binding to the surface of the same cell or inactivated

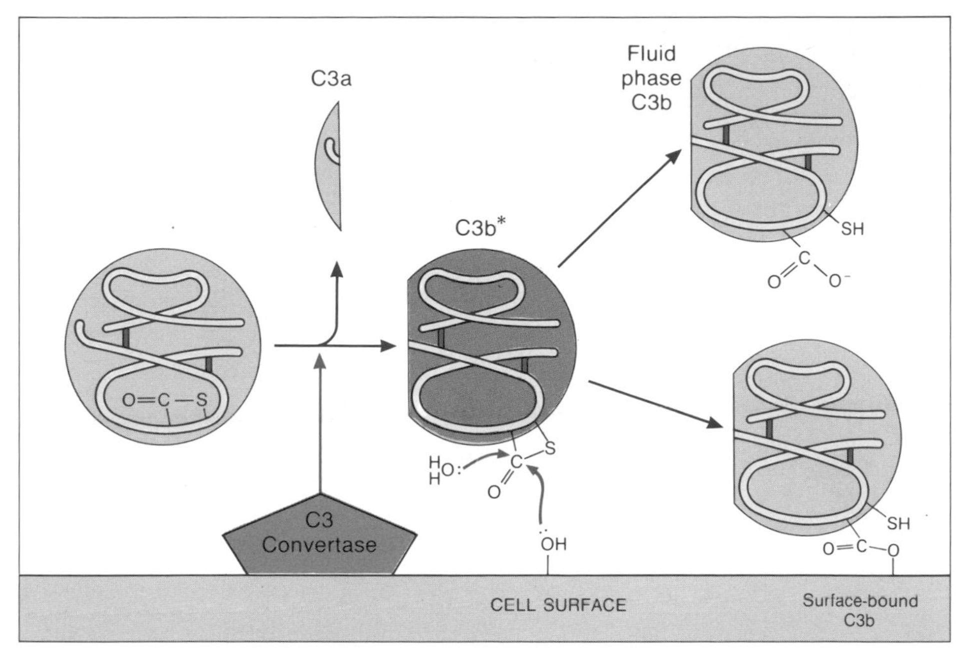

Figure 2.3. Activation of C3. Surface-bound C3-convertase splits the α chain of C3 into C3a and C3b. In the process the internal thiolester in the α chain becomes exposed and C3b is regarded as activated (*). The thiolester either reacts with water to yield fluid phase C3b or with hydroxyl groups on the cell surface to yield surface-bound C3b. C3b* will normally be converted to fluid phase C3b before it can diffuse to neighbouring cells. Interchain disulphide bonds are indicated in solid orange.

by water. The deposition of C3b is minimized on host cells because of their inability to activate the host's own complement pathways.

C4 is a homologue of C3. It also has an internal thiolester and it binds covalently to cell surfaces. However, it differs from C3 in its relative binding efficiencies to amino and hydroxyl groups (see Chapter 3, Sections 3 and 4).

3. Activation of the alternative pathway

Activation of the alternative pathway does not depend upon antibodies recognizing specific molecules on the target cell surface; rather, it relies on molecular structures on the target cell to upset the very delicate balance of proteins involved so that their activation and deposition are focused on its surface.

C3 is continuously activated at a slow rate in the fluid phase by any of the following means: (i) C3 could be cleaved to C3b by serum proteases; (ii) small nucleophiles, or water, could gain access and react with the thiolester (10); (iii) C3 could be subjected to non-specific perturbation leading to a conformational change and the exposure and hydrolysis of the thiolester (13) (*Figure 2.4*). C3

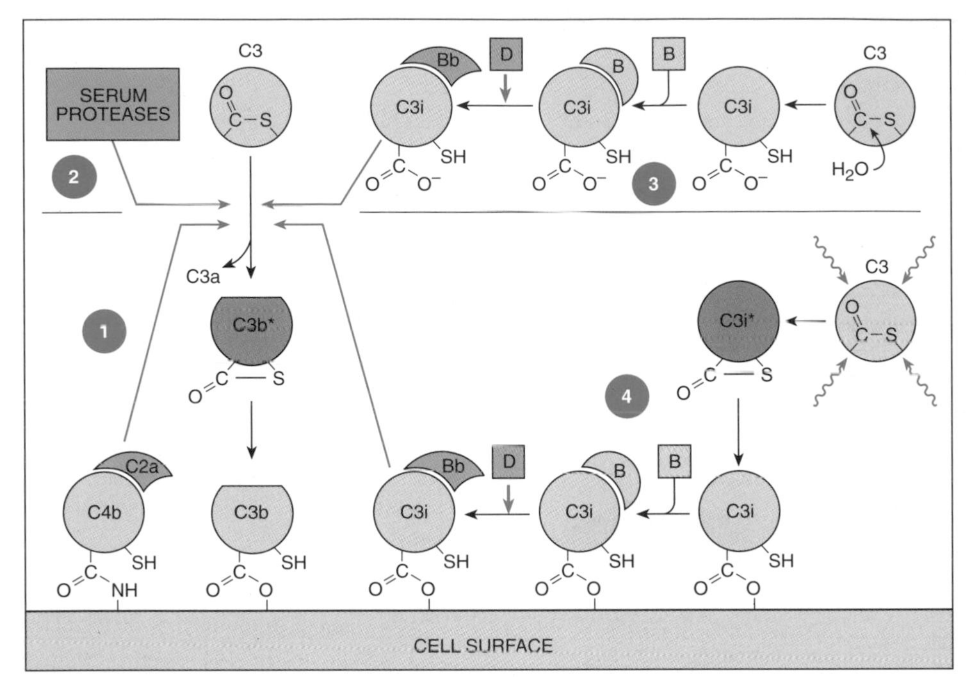

Figure 2.4. The most important mechanism of the initial deposition of C3b on an alternative pathway activator *in vivo* is probably by the C4b2a enzyme of the classical pathway (1). Other mechanisms include cleavage of C3 by serum proteases (2), conversion of C3 into C3i by water or other small nucleophiles (3), and perturbation of the C3 structure, indicated by orange wriggly arrows, leading to the exposure of the thiolester and binding of C3i on to the cell surface (4).

with a hydrolysed thiolester without the loss of its C3a fragment is referred to as C3i, also often designated as C3(H_2O), which has a molecular conformation like C3b and is able to form a C3-convertase with factor B in the presence of factor D (14, 15). It must be stressed that all these processes only operate at low levels, and the probability of covalent deposition of the activated C3b* or C3i* (the * indicates the very short-lived activated molecule) on a cell surface is even lower. However, if a single C3b, or C3i molecule, is deposited on an activating surface of the alternative pathway, it can serve as a seed for the positive amplification loop which operates explosively (16, 17, 18). *In vivo*, both the classical and alternative pathways of complement act in concert to fight against infection, and the most effective mechanism to deposit the initial C3b on a foreign cell surface is by the classical pathway.

It may easily be appreciated that the C3-convertases; $\overline{\text{C3bBb}}$ and $\overline{\text{C3iBb}}$, if left unchecked, would quickly activate all C3 and factor B by a positive feedback mechanism. However, the activation of C3 in the blood, under normal conditions, is kept at a low level by the control proteins factor H and factor I (*Figure 2.5a*). Factor H operates in two ways to inactivate the $\overline{\text{C3bBb}}$ enzyme: (i) it accelerates

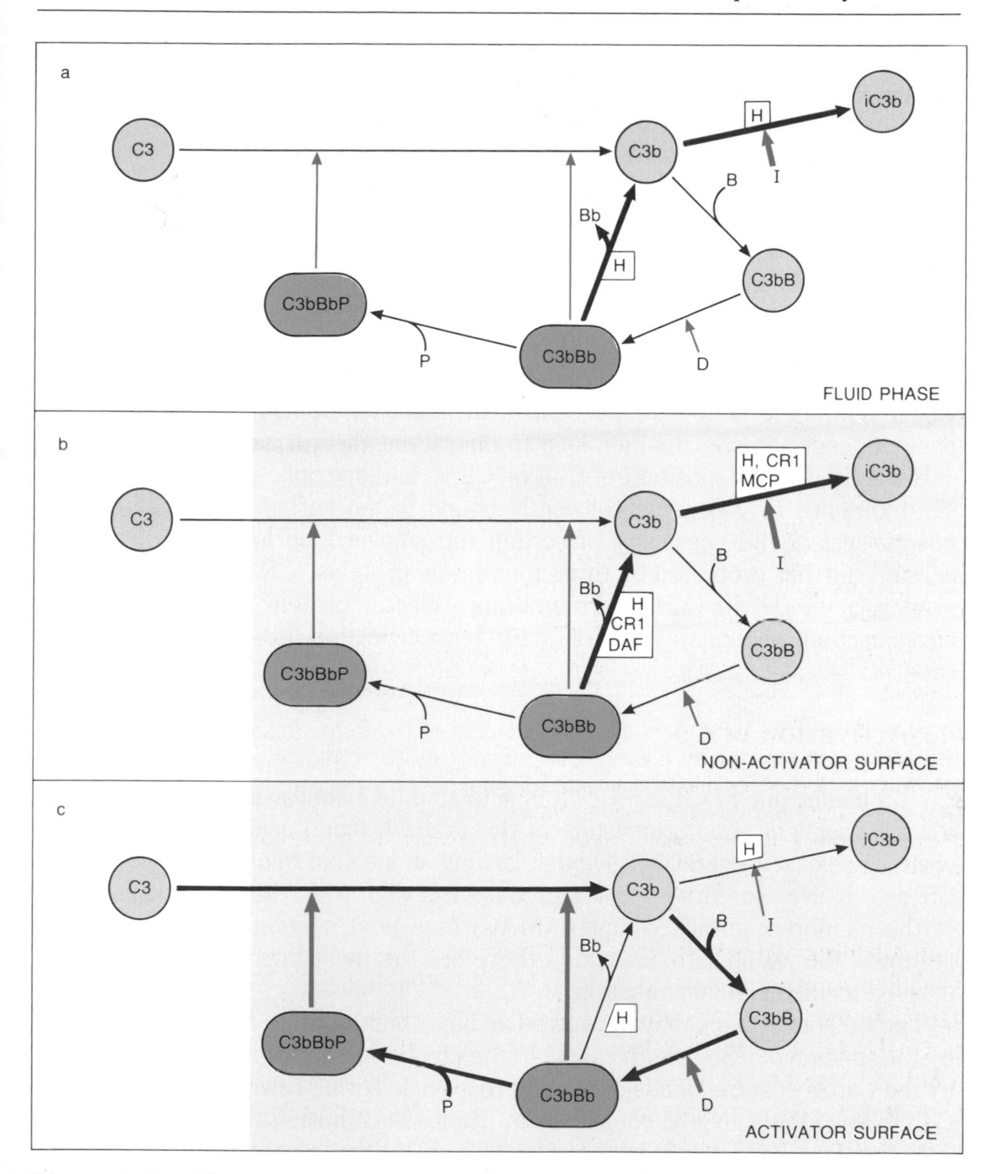

Figure 2.5. The alternative pathway amplification loop is only operative on surfaces where the restriction of C3 conversion by control proteins is deregulated. (**a**) In the fluid phase activation is curtailed by the efficient cleavage of C3b by factor I in the presence of factor H and the efficient dissociation of any C3bBb formed, by factor H. (**b**) Surface-bound C3b on non-activators is regulated similarly as in the fluid phase. In addition to factor H, CR1, DAF, and MCP are also present to further restrict the activation of C3. (**c**) On activator surfaces the regulatory pathways are inhibited and rapid activation of C3 and subsequent deposition of C3b on the surface ensues.

the dissociation of Bb from C3b (19); and (ii) it serves as a cofactor for factor I, a serine protease, which cleaves C3b into iC3b, which can no longer form the C3-convertase with factor B (20). (Individuals with a genetic deficiency of factor I were first diagnosed as being deficient in C3 since their blood C3 level was only about 10% that of normal due to the lack of down regulation of the C3 convertases and the consequent high level of conversion of C3 to C3b.)

A minute amount of C3 activated by schemes 2, 3, and 4 as shown in *Figure 2.4* could be deposited on cell surfaces in a random and non-specific fashion. Non-activating surfaces of the alternative pathway have control proteins to prevent the formation of the $\overline{\text{C3bBb}}$ complex (*Figure 2.5b*). Activating surfaces, however, have the common but undefined property of providing 'protected sites' which retard the action of the control proteins on $\overline{\text{C3bBb}}$, thus allowing the positive feedback C3-activation loop to operate at the surface (*Figure 2.5c*).

Since the initial deposition of C3b or C3i is non-specific, some of the C3b or C3i molecules may become covalently bound to the surface of a host cell. To ensure against the possibility of setting the amplification loop in motion, host cells are further protected by three membrane proteins, CR1 (21), decay accelerating factor (DAF) (22), and membrane cofactor protein (MCP) (23), which have functions similar to those of factor H (see Section 6.3).

4. Activation of C5

C5 is a homologue of C3 and C4. It is activated by a similar mechanism in which a small fragment, C5a, consisting of the first 74 amino acid residues of the α chain, is released from C5b. Though lacking an internal thiolester, activation of C5 also involves conformational change to yield C5b, which initiates the assembly of the membrane attack complex (MAC) (see next section). C5a is the most potent of the anaphylatoxins and is therefore the most important complement-derived mediator in inflammation.

The C5 convertases may be viewed as being built up from the C3-convertases by the addition of C3b in both cases. In the classical pathway, C3, when activated by the $\overline{\text{C4b2a}}$ enzyme, binds covalently to a single serine residue in the α'chain of C4b to form the $\overline{\text{C4b3b2a}}$ complex (24, 25) in which both C4b and C3b serve as cofactors for C2a in the activation of C5 (*Figure 2.6a*). The binding of C5 to C3b is required since C5 is not activated by the $\overline{\text{C4b2a}}$ enzyme. That C5 also needs to bind to C4b came from the study of the C4 allotype C4A6, which has a thiolester, binds covalently to cell surfaces like any other of the C4A allotypes, forms a functional $\overline{\text{C4b2a}}$ complex for C3 activation, and forms a C4b3b covalent complex with C3b (26, 27). However, because of a change of an Arg to a Trp residue in the β chain of C4A6 (28, 29), the final $\overline{\text{C4b3b2a}}$ complex fails to bind, and therefore fails to activate, C5. Similarly, the activation of C3 by the $\overline{\text{C3bBb}}$ enzyme, the C3-convertase of the alternative pathway, leads to the covalent binding of the freshly activated C3b to the C3b of the $\overline{\text{C3bBb}}$ enzyme to give a $\overline{\text{C3b}_2\text{Bb}}$ complex which is the C5-convertase of the alternative pathway (*Figure 2.6b*) (30).

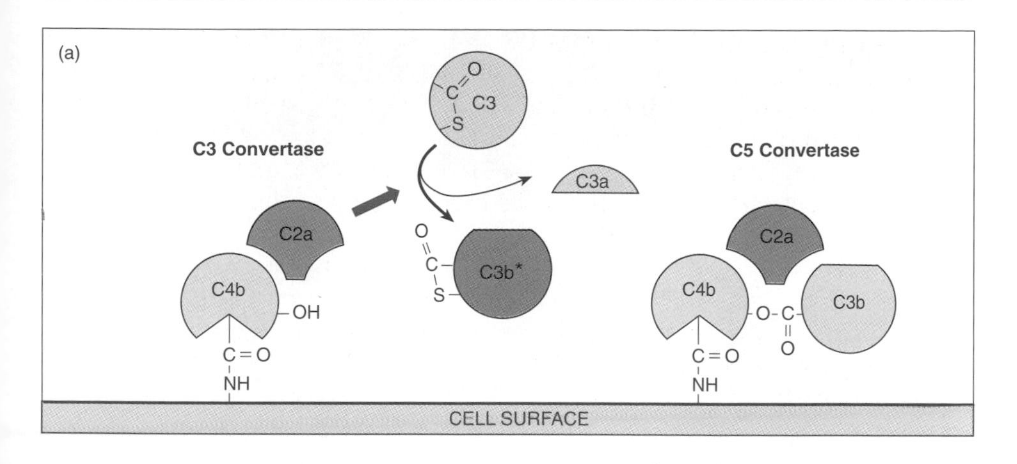

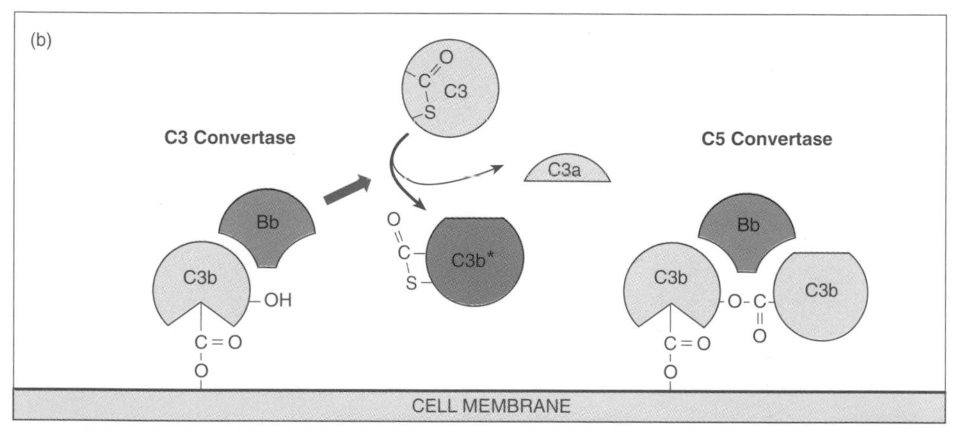

Figure 2.6. The C5 convertases. (a) The classical pathway C5-convertase. Activated C3b* binds to the serine residue at position 1217 of surface-bound C4b to form a C4b–C3b covalent complex, which serves as the cofactor for the catalytic component C2a in the C5-convertase. Note that C4b binds to the cell surface via an amide bond. (b) The alternative pathway C5-convertase. The covalent attachment of a C3b molecule to C3b of the $\overline{\text{C3bBb}}$ complex yields the C5-convertase $\overline{\text{C3b}_2\text{Bb}}$.

5. Activation of the membrane attack complex (MAC) C5b-9

The lytic activity of complement was the first well-defined function attributed to the system and it is now clear that the plasma glycoproteins C5, C6, C7, C8, and C9 undergo a hydrophilic–amphiphilic transition to produce the typical cytolytic complement lesion seen in model systems using red blood cells or liposomes as targets (*Figure 2.7*). It should be noted that C8 is actually a complex of three proteins and the three subunits, α, β, and γ, are distinct gene products. In the heterotrimer, the β subunit is non-covalently associated with the α and γ subunits, which are disulphide-linked. Together the terminal

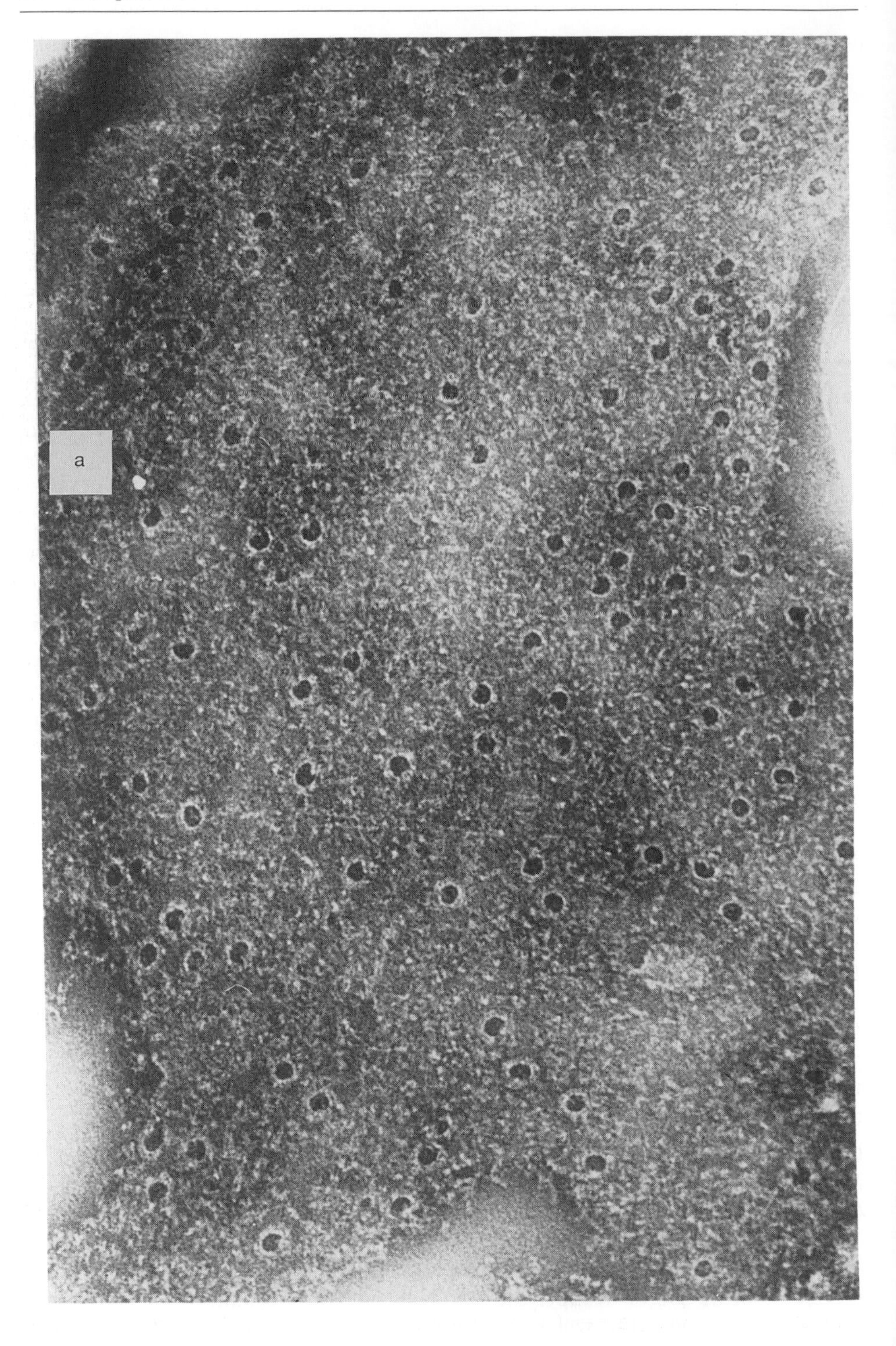
a

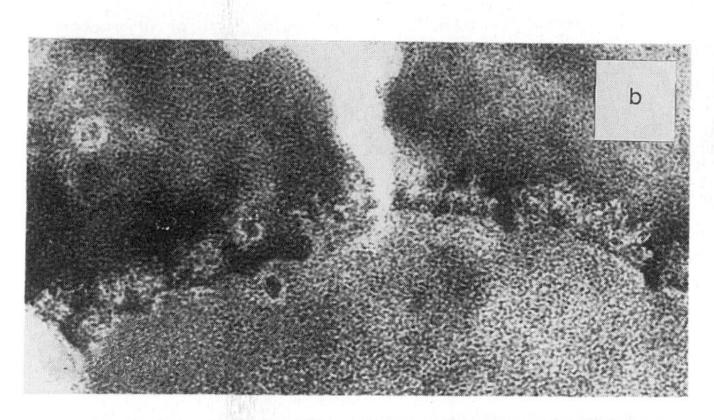

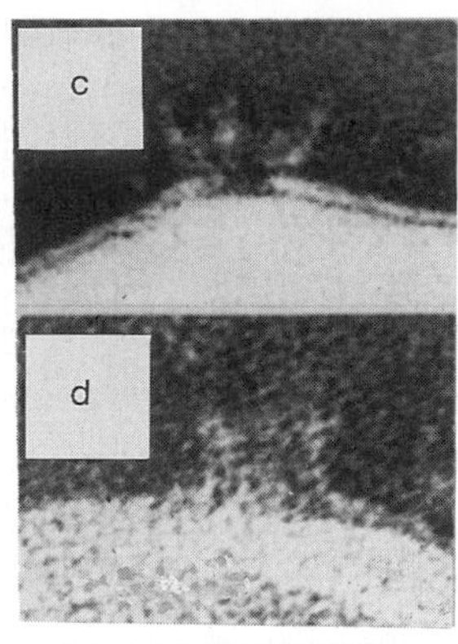

Figure 2.7. (**a**) Electron micrograph of complement lesions formed on an erythrocyte membrane treated with rabbit antibody and guinea pig complement. The lesions are stable and uniform but size (internal diameter of 8.5 to 11 nm) varies with the species of complement used (electron micrograph kindly supplied by Dr E. A. Munn). (**b**) Electron micrograph (from ref. 54 with permission) of complement MAC lesions on lecithin liposomes (artificial membranes) showing lesions in top view, profile, and detached. Higher magnification views of lesions (also from ref. 54) seen in profile from a lecithin liposome (**c**) and from a sphingomyelin cholesterol liposome (**d**).

components, C5 to C9, can produce a complex (M_r 1–2 × 10^6) referred to as the MAC. The MAC forms transmembrane channels which displace lipid molecules and other constituents, thus disrupting the phospholipid bilayer of target cells and allowing the equilibration of small solute molecules across the membrane. An osmotic imbalance is created due to the macromolecules retained inside the cell. The rapid influx of water leads to cell swelling and eventually lysis.

The only proteolytic event in the formation of the MAC is the splitting of C5, to C5a and C5b, by the C5-convertases of either pathway (see *Figure 1.1*). The freshly activated C5b, loosely bound to C3b, binds to C6 to form a C5b-6 complex and then to C7 to form a C5b-7 complex which has a transient binding site for membrane surfaces (*Figure 2.8*) and becomes dissociated from C3b. If the C5b-7 complex fails to bind rapidly to a membrane surface via sites in C6 and C7, its potential cytolytic activity is lost and self-aggregation takes place in the fluid phase. The binding of the three-chain C8 molecule to C5b-7 takes place via a specific C5b recognition site on the β subunit of C8. After C8 is bound the C8α subunit directs the incorporation of C9 to form C5b-9. Although the C5b-8 complex is capable of slowly lysing red blood cells as well as certain nucleated cells, its principal role would appear to be to act as a receptor for C9 and behave as a catalyst in C9 polymerization to yield the highly effective C5b-9 cytolytic complex (*Figure 2.9*). The manner by which C5b-8 binding of one molecule of C9 allows a high affinity C9–C9 interaction is not absolutely clear, but it is likely that the relatively hydrophobic sections of the C-terminal half of C9 become inserted into the phospholipid of the target membrane. The MAC has a composition of C5b-8$(C9)_n$, where n may lie between 1 and 18, but the type of lesion

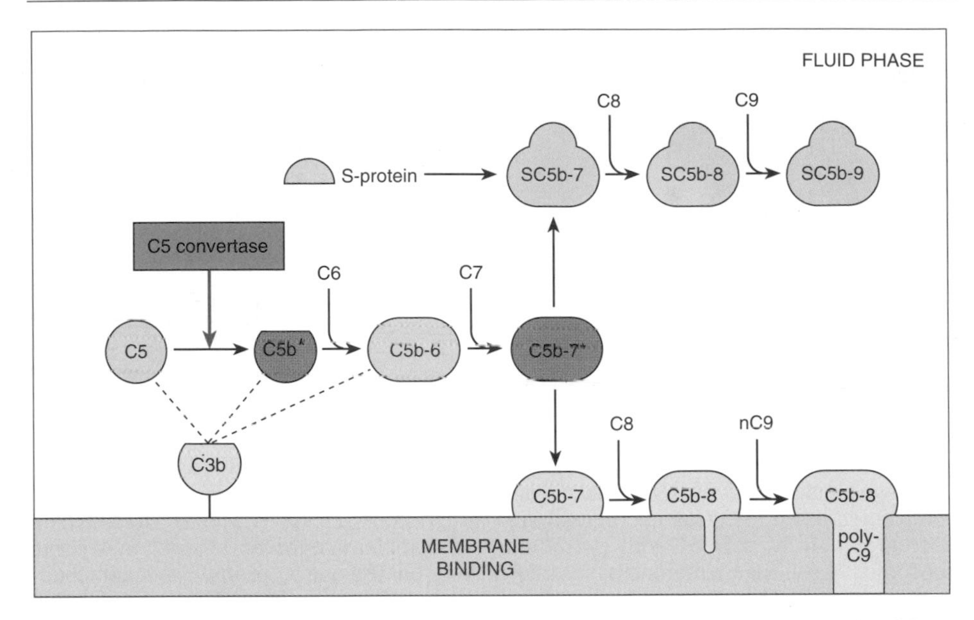

Figure 2.8. Scheme of assembly of the MAC and its control of S-protein. Metastable C5b* and C5b-7* are shaded brown. C5b* and C5b6 are loosely bound to membrane C3b. Initial attachment of the assembling MAC is via a transient binding site in C5b-7.

seen is dependent on the number of C9 molecules (31). In a model system using purified proteins, typical cylinder-like membrane lesions are seen (*Figure 2.7*) at a C9:C5b-8 ratio of 6:1, whereas at a ratio of 1:1 only a network of protein aggregates is seen and no lesions are apparent. However, even at the low C9 input there was efficient cell lysis, indicating that the ring-like lesions may not be a prerequisite for cell lysis and that complexes with a low number of C9 molecules may simply produce smaller, but effective, membrane channels (32, 33).

6. Control of the complement system

Complement is a cascade activation system. The activation steps involving components C1 to C5 in the classical pathway are enzymatic, such that in each step the activation is amplified. Furthermore, the activation of C3 and factor B in the alternative pathway operates in a positive feedback amplification loop (*Figure 2.5*). Thus, in the absence of any control mechanisms, it can be appreciated that the levels of active complement proteins would be reduced rapidly. For example, in the reconstitution of the alternative pathway with only C3, factor B, and factor D, the level of C3 and factor B would quickly be reduced to almost zero by the uncontrolled activity of the $\overline{C3bBb}$ complex.

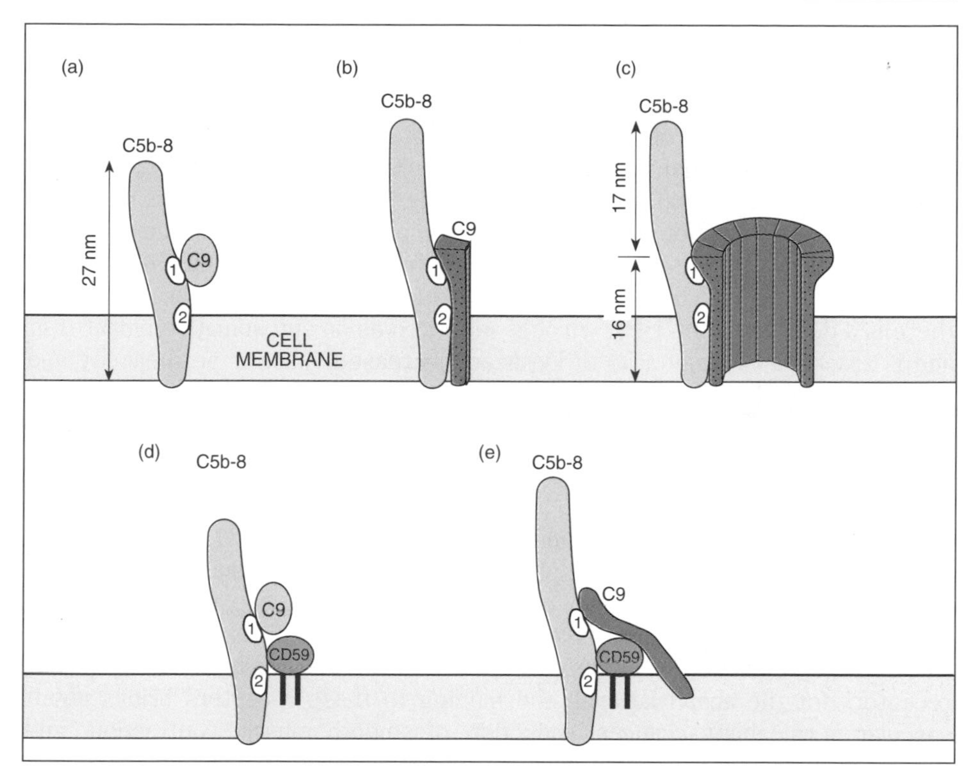

Figure 2.9. Formation of poly-C9 directed by C5b-8. Initial binding of C9 to site 1 of C5b-8 (**a**) is reversible. A conformational change in C9 promotes its irreversible binding to site 2 (**b**). Binding of additional C9 leads to their polymerization and the formation of the MAC (**c**). CD59 binds to a site on C5b-8 (**d**) such that the binding of C9 to site 2 and the subsequent formation of MAC is blocked (**e**). (Adapted from refs 49 and 55.)

The activated components of the pathways come under the control of various regulatory proteins and enzymes as discussed in Sections 6.1–6.5. In addition, it should be noted that the C3 and C5 convertases decay quite rapidly by the dissociation of the enzymatic components C2a and factor Bb from the cofactor components in the absence of control proteins, and that C4b, C3b, and C5b-7 display only transient ability to bind to target surfaces.

6.1 C1-inhibitor (C1-Inh) and the C1 complex

After activation of C1 has taken place, for example by its binding to immune complexes, the C1-Inh rapidly forms a covalent 1:1 complex with both the activated C1r and C1s, probably via the catalytic sites, resulting in the release of the (C1-Inh)–C1r–C1s–(C1-Inh) complexes (34). This prevents over-activation of the classical pathway and efficiently removes $C\overline{1r}$ and $C\overline{1s}$ from the activator–C1 complex, thus leaving the collagen-like regions of C1q to interact with the widespread C1q receptor and fulfil a number of effector functions which include cell-mediated cytotoxicity, inhibition of interleukin-1 production, stimulation of oxidative metabolism in polymorphonuclear leukocytes, and Fc-receptor-mediated phagocytosis.

C1-Inh is a member of the serpin family of inhibitors (35) and, although it inhibits a variety of other activated plasma proteases (including kallikrein, plasmin, Hageman factor, and factor XI), it is likely that its major role lies in control of complement activation since it is the only plasma inhibitor directed against $C\overline{1r}$ and $C\overline{1s}$ (34). The importance of C1-Inh is illustrated from the study of patients suffering from hereditary angioneurotic oedema (HANE) (36). In HANE there is a deficiency of C1-Inh which is inherited as an autosomal dominant trait and is associated with attacks of localized, increased vascular permeability and it is suspected that the kinin-like activity in the disease may emanate from an over-activation of C2 and/or bradykinin.

6.2 Anaphylatoxin inactivator

The anaphylatoxins C3a, C4a, and C5a are all peptides, 74–77 amino acid residues long, released from the splitting of a single Arg–X bond in the α chains of C3, C4, and C5 respectively upon activation of the complement system. These peptides mediate many inflammatory responses and have also been implicated in the regulation of immune responses (37). A variety of cells possess receptors for the anaphylatoxins and binding to these receptors brings about vascular permeability changes, induction of smooth muscle contraction, and release of histamine from mast cells and basophils. The spasmogenic activities of the three anaphylatoxins are in the order of C5a $>$ C3a $>$ C4a. These activities are controlled in the blood by the anaphylatoxin inactivator (serum carboxypeptidase N), which can remove the C-terminal Arg from each of the anaphylatoxins and render them inactive. C5a also mediates an additional set of neutrophil stimulatory activities, including chemotaxis and superoxide production, by interacting with a receptor coupled to a GTP-binding protein complex. The removal of the C-terminal Arg of C5a does not appear to affect its neutrophil stimulatory activities. Thus, C5a is probably the most important of the anaphylatoxins in terms of normal host defence mechanisms.

6.3 Factor I and its cofactors and related regulatory proteins

Factor I is a highly specific serine protease which is involved with the regulation of the C3/C5-convertases of either pathway. Using C4-binding protein (C4bp) or H as cofactors it splits the α' chains of C4b or C3b, respectively, causing rapid loss of the biological activities associated with C4b and C3b, which includes their roles in the C3/C5-convertases. Two membrane proteins, the complement receptor type 1 (CR1) and the membrane cofactor protein (MCP), can also serve as cofactors for factor I in the cleavage of C3b and C4b. Unlike C4bp and H, the two membrane proteins can serve as cofactors for both C3b and also the C4b cleavage reactions (38).

Other than serving as cofactor for factor I in the cleavage of C3b and C4b, the regulatory proteins also accelerate the decay of the C3/C5-convertase complexes. The formation of the classical C3-convertase, for example, involves the initial interaction between C4b and native C2, which becomes sensitive to C1 cleavage into C2a and C2b. Under normal conditions, and in the absence of other proteins, the C2a remains bound to C4b as the $\overline{C4b2a}$ complex only for a limited period, in the order of 1–5 min, after which C2a is dissociated from C4b resulting in the loss of C3-convertase activity. Another C2 molecule may bind to the same C4b and the formation of a new $\overline{C4b2a}$ complex may take place. The regulatory protein C4bp can accelerate the dissociation of C2a from C4b. Factor H, CR1, and the membrane bound decay acceleration factor (DAF) mediate similar activity on their respective substrate complexes.

The five regulatory proteins are related structurally since they are constructed almost exclusively with CCP (complement control protein) domains (see Chapter 3, Section 5). Their overlapping regulatory roles on C3b, C4b, and the C3/C5-convertase complexes are best illustrated in *Table 2.1*. Whereas the soluble proteins factor H and C4bp can mediate both decay acceleration and cofactor activity specific for C3b and C4b, respectively, the membrane bound proteins MCP and DAF mediate only one of the two regulatory activities, as their names imply, but are indiscriminate with respect to C3b and C4b. It should be noted that CR1 mediates all four activities in addition to serving as a receptor for C3b and C4b (39).

Factor I cleaves C3b at two positions in the α′ chain to yield iC3b and C3f (40). iC3b is further degraded by various serum proteases to C3c, C3dg, and C3d (*Figure 2.10*). While iC3b, C3dg, and C3d do not play any role in complement activation, they are important as ligands for the receptors CR3 (for iC3b) and CR2 (for iC3b, C3dg, and C3d). The interaction of C3 fragments, i.e. C3b, iC3b, C3dg, and C3d, on immune complexes or target cells with C3 receptors on host leukocytes as well as erythrocytes and platelets is important for the clearance of the immune complexes and the stimulation of immune response. Factor I cleaves two sites on the α′ chain of C4b on either side of the

Table 2.1 Inhibitory activities of the regulators of complement activation protein family

Proteins	Dissociation of C3 and C5 convertases		Cofactor for Factor I cleavage of	
	Classical $\overline{C4b2a}$ and $\overline{C4b3b2a}$	Alternative $\overline{C3bBb}$ and $\overline{C3b_2Bb}$	C4b	C3b
C4bp	+	–	+	–
Factor H	–	+	–	+
DAF	+	+	–	–
MCP	–	–	+	+
CR1	+	+	+	+

Adapted from ref. 39.

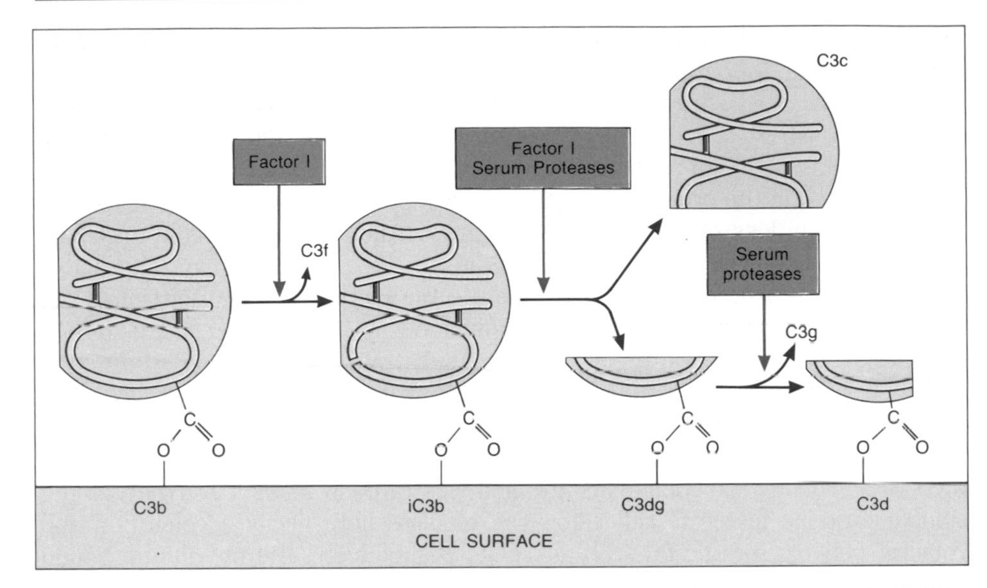

Figure 2.10. Breakdown of C3b. (1) Surface-bound C3b with an α′ chain of 103 kDa and a β chain of 75 kDa is cleaved by factor I, in the presence of cofactors, at two places on the α′ chain to release C3f (3 kDa), leaving the α′ chain in two fragments of 60 kDa (N-terminal) and 40 kDa (C-terminal). (2) Serum proteases or factor I in association with CR1 cleave the 60 kDa fragment into two fragments of 23 kDa (N-terminal) and 37 kDa (C3dg). The released C3c thus contains three chains including an intact β chain and two fragments, derived from the α′ chain, of 23 kDa and 40 kDa. (3) Addition of exogenous proteases to surface-bound C3dg results in the release of C3g (5 kDa) leaving C3d (32 kDa) on the cell surface. Interchain disulphide bonds are indicated in solid orange.

thiolester to yield C4c and C4d (41). It is not known if C3c, C3f, and C4c mediate any biological activities, and C4d does not appear to be a ligand of any receptor.

6.4 Regulation of the membrane attack complex

A number of proteins, both in the fluid phase and membrane bound, are found to have an inhibitory effect on the lytic activity of the MAC. The fluid phase inhibitory proteins bind to the various intermediates of MAC, notably the C5b-7 complex, which has a transient binding site for the lipid bilayers, when they diffuse away from the target cell on which they are activated and may bind to bystander host cells. Binding of the C5b-7 complex to the control proteins abolishes their capacity to bind to membranes. The most prominent member of the soluble inhibitory protein in the S-protein, a serum protein of M_r 80 000 Da which was invariably found in MAC purified from activated sera (*Figure 2.8*). Up to three molecules of S-protein can bind to the C5b-7 complex and it has been identified as the 'spreading protein' vitronectin (42, 43). Other serum lipoproteins including the apolipoprotein SP40,40 (also known as clusterin) can also inhibit the C5b-7 activity by similar mechanisms (44, 45). SP40,40 is found at high concentrations in seminal plasma, and may have a role in protecting spermatozoa from complement attack (46, 47).

It has been a long-standing observation that the MAC is more effective in lysing heterologous rather than autologous red blood cells and this phenomenon appears to be related to the presence of two membrane proteins of the host cells. A protein of M_r 65 000 Da had been called the 'C8 binding protein', 'MAC-inhibiting factor', or the 'homologous restriction factor'. As the name implies, this protein binds to C8 and interferes with the subsequent assembly of the MAC (48). A smaller protein of M_r 19 000 Da also has homologous restriction activity. This protein has been identified as the surface antigen CD59 but has also been known as an homologous restriction factor (HRF20) or a MAC-inhibiting factor (MACIF). It binds to the C5b-8 complex, and although it does not appear to inhibit the binding of the first C9 molecule on C5b-8, it prevents the conformational change of C9 required for the binding of additional C9 and their subsequent polymerization (*Figure 2.9*) (49). CD59 has a GPI anchor and it is present on the membrane of many cells and tissues. CD59 has also been found in the prostasomes of seminal plasma. It is postulated that the partition of CD59 from prostasomes to spermatozoa may confer the latter with MAC resistance (50).

6.5 The stabilizing role of properdin

Properdin was the first of the alternative pathway proteins to be identified, with the result that the alternative pathway was, and sometimes still is, referred to as the 'properdin' pathway. It is present in plasma in the form of a mixture of cyclic polymers, predominantly tetramers and trimers (51). The monomer (M_r 56 000 Da) appears highly asymmetric when viewed in the electron microscope (26 nm × 3 nm) and it associates in a head-to-tail fashion to form the polymers (*Figure 2.11*). Properdin is, to date, the only control protein in normal plasma which displays a stabilizing rather than a disruptive or degradative role. It does this by binding to C3b in the $\overline{C3bBb}$ complex thus significantly increasing the life of the C3/C5-convertases.

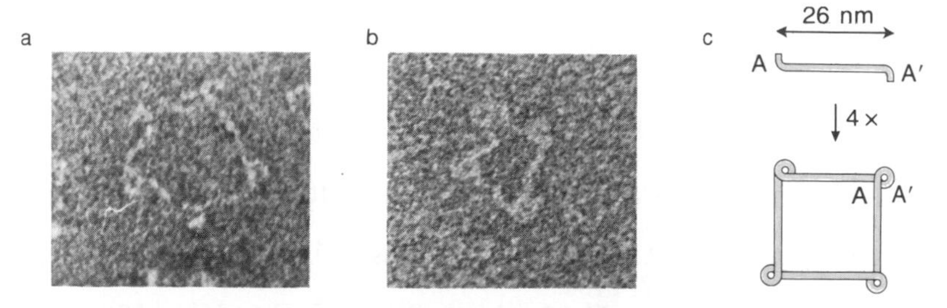

Figure 2.11. Electron micrographs of properdin oligomers (from ref. 51 with permission): (**a**) cyclic pentamer, and (**b**) cyclic tetramer. Magnification is × 320 000. The dimension of a monomer was estimated to be about 26 nm in length and 3 nm in width. (**c**) A model for a cyclic tetramer is shown where complementary binding sites (A and A′) are localized at ends of the monomeric properdin.

7. Further reading

7.1 C1 activation

Arlaud,G.J., Colomb,M.G., and Gagnon,J. (1987). *Immunol. Today*, **8,** 106.
Schumaker,V.N., Zavodsky,P., and Poon,P.H. (1987). *Annu. Rev. Immunol.*, **5,** 21.
Behring Inst. Mitt. (1993). **93,** Entire volume.

7.2 Activation of the complement pathways

Holmskov,U., Malhotra,R., Sim,R.B., and Jensenius,J.C. (1994). *Immunol. Today*, **15,** 67.
Lachmann,P.J. and Hughes-Jones,N.C. (1985). In *Complement* (ed. H.J.Müller-Eberhard and P.A.Meischer), p. 147. Springer, Berlin.
Pangburn,M.K. (1986). In *Immunobiology of the complement system* (ed. G.D.Ross), p. 45. Academic Press, New York.
Reid,K.B.M. (1986). *Essays Biochem.*, **22**, 27.

7.3 Internal thiolester and covalent binding of C3

Law,S.K.A. (1983). *Ann. N.Y. Acad. Sci.*, **421,** 246.
Levine,R.P. and Dodds,A.W. (1989). *Current Topics Microbiol. Immunol*, **153,** 73.
Tack,B.F. (1985). In *Complement* (ed. H.J.Müller-Eberhard and P.A.Miescher), p. 49. Springer, Berlin.

7.4 Membrane attack complex

Müller-Eberhard,H.J. (1986). *Annu. Rev. Immunol.*, **4,** 503.
Podack,E.R. (1986). In *Immunobiology of the complement system* (ed. G.D.Ross), p. 115. Academic Press, New York.

8. References

1. Reid,K.B.M. (1983). *Biochem. Soc. Trans.*, **11,** 1.
2. Gewurz,H., Ying,S.C., Jiang,H., and Lint,T.E. (1993). *Behring Inst. Mitt.*, **93,** 138.
3. Sim,R.B. and Reboul,A. (1981). *Meth. Enzymol.*, **80,** 43.
4. Kilpatrick,J.M. and Volanakis,J.E. (1991). *Immunol. Res.*, **10,** 43.
5. Ji,Y-H, Fujita,T., Hatsuse,H., Takahasi,A., Matsushita,M., and Kawakami,M. (1993). *J. Immunol.*, **150,** 571.
6. Lu,J., Thiel,S., Widemann,H., Timpl,R., and Reid,K.B.M. (1990). *J. Immunol.*, **144,** 2287.
7. Super,M., Thiel,S., Lu,J., Levinsky,R.J., and Turner,M.W. (1989). *Lancet*, **2,** 1236.
8. Müller-Eberhard,H.J., Dalmasso,A.P., and Calcott,M.A. (1966). *J. Exp. Med.*, **124,** 33.
9. Tack,B.F., Harrison,R.A., Janatova,J., Thomas,M.L., and Prahl,J.W. (1980). *Proc. Natl Acad. Sci. USA*, **77,** 5764.
10. Pangburn,M.K. and Müller-Eberhard,H.J. (1980). *J. Exp. Med.*, **152,** 1102.
11. Law,S.K. and Levine,R.P. (1977). *Proc. Natl Acad. Sci. USA*, **74,** 2701.
12. Law,S.K., Lichtenberg,N.A., and Levine,R.P. (1979). *J. Immunol.*, **123,** 1388.
13. Law,S.K.A. (1983). *Biochem. J.*, **211,** 381.
14. Pangburn,M.K., Schreiber,R.D., and Müller-Eberhard,H.J. (1981). *J. Exp. Med.* **154,** 856.

15. Isenman,D.E., Kells,D.I.C., Cooper,N.R., Müller-Eberhard,H.J., and Pangburn,M.K. (1981). *Biochemistry*, **20**, 4458.
16. Nicol,P.A.E. and Lachmann,P.J. (1973). *Immunology*, **24**, 259.
17. Fearon,D.T. and Austen,K.F. (1977). *J. Exp. Med.*, **146**, 22.
18. Pangburn,M.K. and Müller-Eberhard,H.J. (1978). *Proc. Natl Acad. Sci. USA*, **75**, 2416.
19. Whaley,K. and Ruddy,S. (1976). *Science*, **193**, 1011.
20. Pangburn,M.K., Schreiber,R.D., and Müller-Eberhard,H.J. (1977). *J. Exp. Med.*, **146**, 257.
21. Fearon,D.T. (1979). *Proc. Natl Acad. Sci. USA*, **76**, 5867.
22. Nicholson-Weller,A., Burge,J., Fearon,D.T., Weller,P.F., and Austen,K.F. (1982). *J. Immunol.*, **129**, 184.
23. Seya,T., Turner,J.R., and Atkinson,J.P. (1986). *J. Exp. Med.*, **163**, 837.
24. Takata,Y., Kinoshita,T., Kozono,H., Takeda,J., Tanaka,E., Hong,K., and Inoue,K. (1987). *J. Exp. Med.*, **165**, 1494.
25. Kim,Y.U., Carroll,M.C., Isenman,D.E., Nonaka,M., Pramoonjago,P., Takeda,J., Inoue,K., and Kinoshita,T. (1992). *J. Biol. Chem.*, **267**, 4171.
26. Dodds,A.W., Law,S.K.A., and Porter,R.R. (1985). *EMBO J.*, **4**, 2239.
27. Kinoshita,T., Dodds,A.W., Law,S.K.A., and Inoue,K. (1989). *Biochem. J.*, **261**, 743.
28. Anderson,M.J., Milner,C.M., Cotton,R.G.H., and Campbell,R.D. (1992). *J. Immunol.*, **148**, 2795.
29. Ebanks,R.O., Jaikaran,A.S.I., Carroll,M.C., Anderson,M.J., Campbell,R.D., and Isenman,D.E. (1992). *J. Immunol.*, **148**, 2803.
30. Kinoshita,T., Takata,Y., Kozono,H., Takeda,J., Hong,K., and Inoue,K. (1988). *J. Immunol.*, **141**, 3895.
31. Podack,E.R., Tschopp,J., and Müller-Eberhard,H.J. (1982). *J. Exp. Med.*, **156**, 268.
32. Bhakdi,S. and Tranum-Jenson,J. (1986). *J. Immunol.*, **136**, 2999.
33. Dankert,J.R. and Esser,A.F. (1985). *Proc. Natl Acad. Sci. USA*, **82**, 2128.
34. Sim,R.B. and Reboul,A. (1981). *Meth. Enzymol.*, **80**, 43.
35. Bock,S.C., Skriver,K., Nielsen,E., Thogersen,H-C., Wiman,B., Donaldson,V.H., Eddy,R.L., Marrinan,J., Radziejewski,R., Huber,R., Shows,T.B., and Magnusson,S. (1986). *Biochemistry*, **25**, 4292.
36. Donaldson,V.H., Harrison,R.A., Rosen,F.S., Bing,D.H., Kindness,G., Canar,J., Wagner,C.G., and Awad,S. (1985). *J. Clin. Invest.*, **75**, 124.
37. Hugli,T.E. (1981). *CRC Crit. Rev. Immunol.*, **1**, 321.
38. Law,S.K.A. (1988). *J. Cell Sci.*, **9** (Suppl.), 67.
39. Weisman,H.F., Bartow,T., Leppo,M.K., Marsh,H.C., Jr., Carson,G.R., Concino,M.F., Boyle,M.P., Roux,K.H., Weisfeldt,M.L., and Fearon,D.T. (1990). *Science*, **149**, 146.
40. Harrison,R.A. and Lachmann,P.J. (1980). *Mol. Immunol.*, **17**, 9.
41. Fujita,T. and Nussenzweig,V. (1979). *J. Exp. Med.*, **150**, 267.
42. Kolb,W.P. and Müller-Eberhard,H.J. (1975). *J. Exp. Med.*, **141**, 724.
43. Jenne,D. and Stanley,K.K. (1985) *EMBO J.*, **4**, 3153.
44. Murphy,B.F., Kirszbaum,L., Walker,I.D., and d'Apice,A.J.F. (1988). *J. Clin. Invest.*, **81**, 1858.
45. Hamilton,K.K., Zhao,J., and Sims,P.J. (1993). *J. Biol. Chem.*, **268**, 3632.
46. Jenne,D.E. and Tschopp,J. (1989). *Proc. Natl Acad. Sci. USA*, **86**, 7123.
47. O'Bryan, M.K., Baker,H.W.G., Saunders,J.R., Kirszbaum,L., Walker,I.D., Hudson,P., Liu,D.Y., Glew,M.D., d'Apice,A.J.F., and Murphy,B.F. (1990). *J. Clin. Invest.*, **85**, 1477.
48. Zalman,L.S., Wood,L.M., and Müller-Eberhard,H.J. (1986). *Proc. Natl Acad. Sci. USA*, **83**, 6975.
49. Lachmann,P.J. (1991). *Immunol. Today*, **12**, 312.

50. Rooney,I.A., Atkinson,J.P., Krul,E.S., Schonfeld,G., Polakoski,K. Saffitz,J.E., and Morgan,B.P. (1993). *J. Exp. Med.*, **177**, 1409.
51. Smith,C.A., Pangburn,M.K., Vogel,C.W., and Müller-Eberhard,H.J. (1984). *J. Biol. Chem.*, **259**, 4582.
52. Knobel,H.R., Villiger,W., and Isliker,H. (1975). *Eur. J. Immunol.*, **5**, 78.
53. Arlaud,G.J., Colomb,M.G., and Gagnon,J. (1987). *Immunol. Today*, **8**, 106.
54. Lachmann,P.J., Bowyer, Nicol,P., Dawson,R.M.C., and Munn,E.A. (1973). *Immunology*, **24**, 135.
55. Podack,E.R., Preissner,K.T., and Müller-Eberhard,H.J. (1984). *Acta Pathol. Microbiol. Scand.*, Series C **92** (Suppl. 248), 89.

3

Groups and families of proteins in the complement system

As the primary structures of more proteins become available, it is clear that many of them are constructed from modular units. These units have recognizable sequence features and are usually assigned the name of one of the first proteins in which they were fully described. For example, the immunoglobulin (Ig) domains, the epidermal growth factor (EGF) domains, and the complement control protein (CCP) domains are found in many proteins in addition to those from which their names derived. In the cases where the three-dimensional structure of a particular type of modular unit is known, the proteins containing this type of modular unit may be modelled accordingly. The complement proteins mediate a very complex set of activities requiring them to interact with each other as well as molecules present on various cell surfaces and tissues. It is therefore not surprising that they are a diverse group of proteins with mixed evolutionary origins. Some of them are composites of many different types of modules. In this chapter, we describe the complement proteins under an arbitrary set of headings with the aim of illustrating their functions, structures, evolutionary origins, and their relationships to each other as well as to proteins outside the complement system.

1. C1q and related proteins

C1q has an unusual modular structure (1) consisting of collagen-like triple-helical regions connected to globular 'head' regions (*Figure 3.1*, see also *Figure 2.1*). The members of a family of mammalian lectins, containing collagen-like structures, all show a strong overall structural similarity to C1q. These carbohydrate-binding proteins belong to the group III of the family of Ca^{2+}-dependent, C-type lectins and include three plasma proteins (mannan binding protein, MBP; conglutinin; and collectin-43) and two lung surfactant proteins (SP-A and SP-D) (2). They have been defined as the 'collectins' i.e. *co*llagen-like *lectins*. Like C1q, each of the collectins is a macromolecule which contains 12 to 18 polypeptide chains

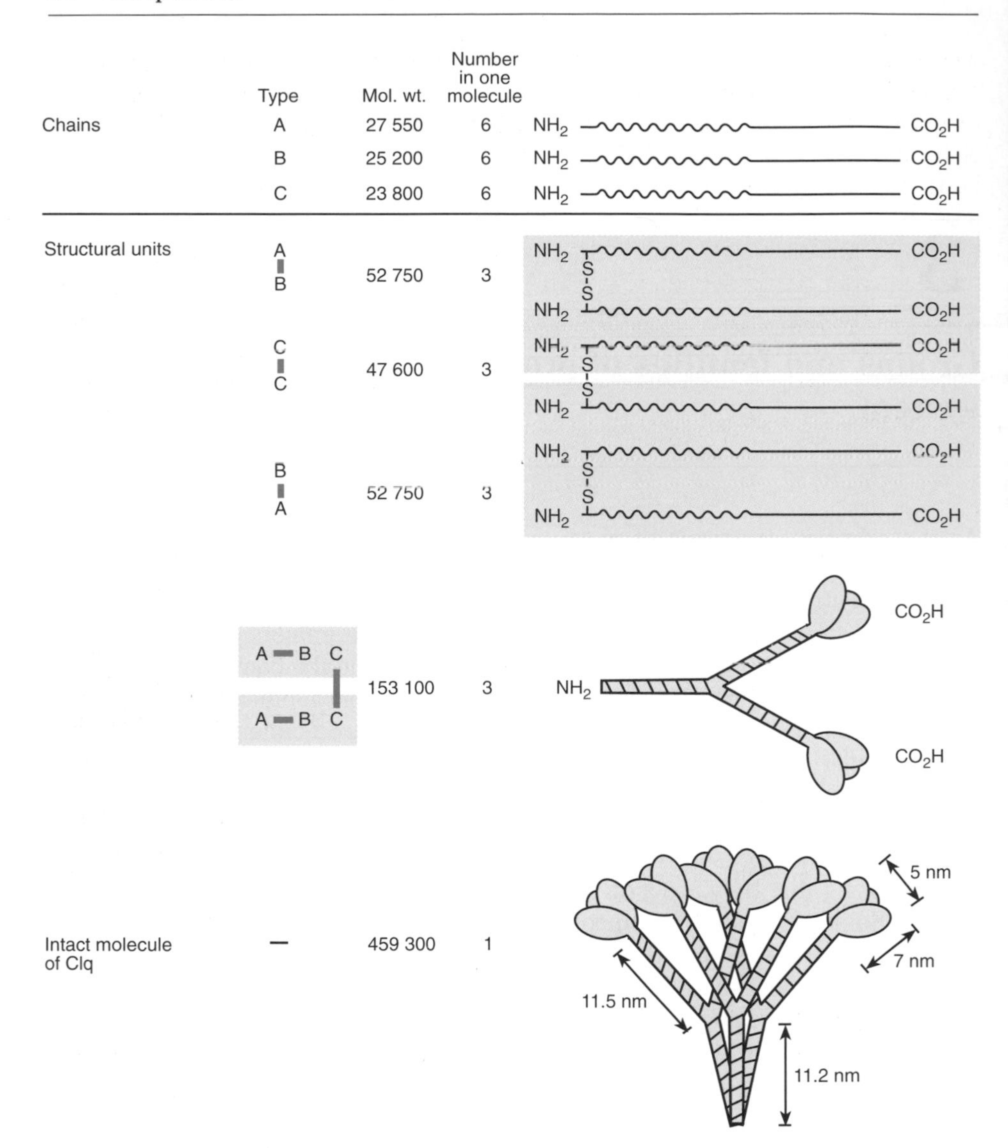

Figure 3.1. A molecular model of C1q. ~~~~ and ▭▭▭ denote collagen-like amino acid sequence and triple-helical structure respectively. The molecule consists of 18 chains with the N-terminal portions of the A, B, or C chains having collagen-like sequences which adopt a triple-helical structure. Each of the six globular 'heads' contains one each of the C-terminal portion of the A, B, and C chains, thus each head is shown as a composite of three subunits. The A and B chains are disulphide bonded at the N-terminal region. The C chain is disulphide bonded to the C chain of another monomeric ABC subunit. Three dimeric subunits are held by non-covalent forces to give the hexameric structure of C1q. The C1r and C1s binding sites are located in the collagen region whereas the binding sites for the Fc regions of IgG or IgM are in the globular heads.

which have their amino acid sequences organized into N-terminal collagen-like regions and C-terminal 'globular' regions. However, it should be emphasized that C1q does not contain C-type carbohydrate recognition domains in its globular 'heads'. The C1q 'heads' are known to bind to peptide sequences in the Fc regions of IgG (C_H2) and IgM (C_H3) rather than to carbohydrate structures, where IgG(C_H2) and IgM(C_H3) are the second and third constant domains of the heavy chains of IgG and IgM respectively. The C1q globular modules are related in amino acid sequence (around 23% identity) to sequences found in the C-terminal globular portions of the type VIII and type X collagens. The genes encoding the A, B, and C chains of human C1q and the α chain of type VIII collagen are located on chromosome 1 (1p 34.1–36.3 and 1p 32.3–34.3 respectively) while those encoding MBP, SP-A, and SP-D are found in a cluster on human chromosome 10 (10q 21–23).

1.1 C1q

The C1q molecule contains 18 polypeptide chains (six A, six B, and six C) with each of the three types of chain containing a region of 81 amino acids of a collagen-like (-Gly-Xaa-Yaa-)$_n$ repeating sequence starting close to the N-terminal end and which is followed by a C-terminal portion of about 136 amino acids which are non-collagen-like (1). Triple helical structures are formed between the collagen-like regions of one each of the A, B, and C chains, while the globular 'head' regions are formed between the non-collagen-like regions. Thus, one C1q molecule is composed of six triple helices which are aligned in parallel throughout half their length and then diverge for the remainder of their length of triple helical structure to form the connecting strands, each of which extends into one of the six globular 'head' regions (*Figure 3.1*). The collagen-like connecting strands interact with the $C1r_2$–$C1s_2$ tetramer to give the C1 complex which, after activation, splits and activates C4 and C2.

1.2 Mannan binding protein (MBP) and conglutinin

Two of the collectins (MBP and conglutinin) interact directly with complement components and most of the collectins appear to bind, via their collagen-like regions, to the cell-surface C1q receptor (2). MBP, like C1q, is found in a hexameric form having six globular 'heads' each attached to collagen-like 'tails' (*Figure 3.2a*) but, unlike C1q which is always found in a hexameric form, MBP can be isolated in the form of dimers, trimers, tetramers, and pentamers (*Figure 3.2a*). In addition, the monomeric unit of human serum MBP is composed of three copies of the same chain, thus a hexamer would have 18 identical chains. However, only the MBP hexamers appear efficient at interacting with pro-enzymes $C1r_2$–$C1s_2$ and bringing about activation after their binding to suitable carbohydrate ligands. Recently a new serum protease, designated 'MBP-associated serine protease' or 'MASP', has been described (3, 4, 5) which interacts with MBP. The interaction of MBP with carbohydrate ligands can cause the activation of the pro-enzyme form of MASP and it may be that MASP, rather than $C1r_2$–

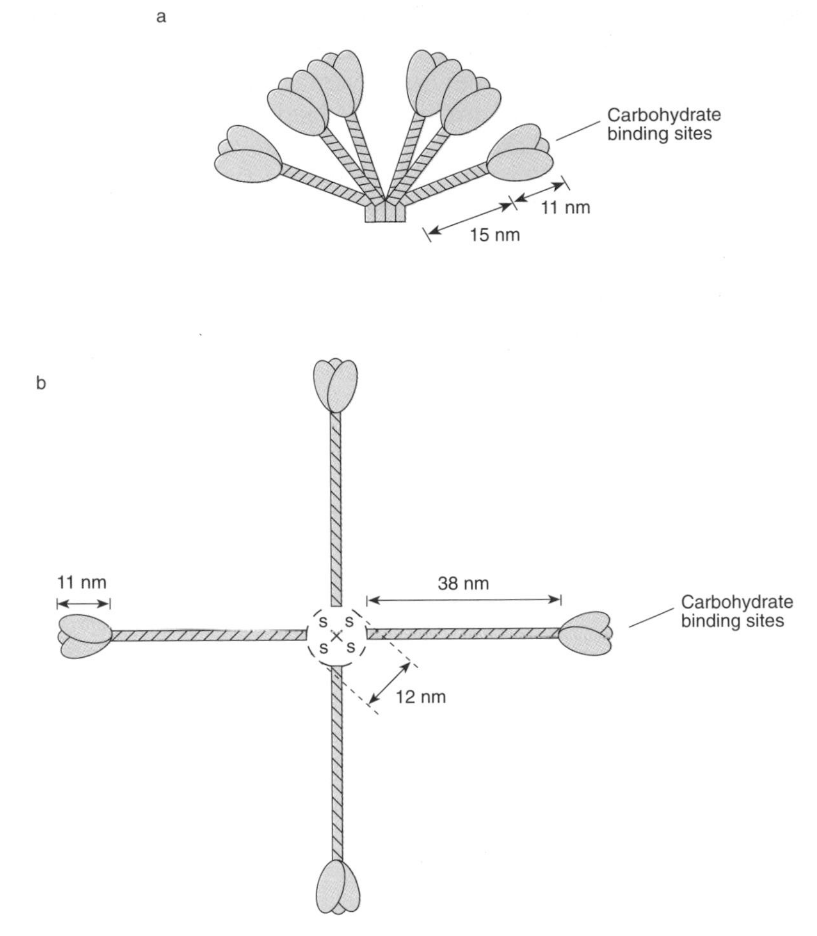

Figure 3.2. (**a**) A side view of the hexameric form of human serum MBP. [hatched bar] denotes triple-helical structure. In contrast to C1q, the three chains in each monomeric subunit are identical. Each head of MPB contains three C-type lectin domains. The electron micrographs are from ref. 115 and show tetramer, pentamer, and hexamer forms of the molecule. In blood the hexamer form is considered as being the natural form of the molecule which is involved in complement activation. (**b**) A model for bovine conglutinin. [hatched bar] denotes triple-helical structure. Each of the four 'head' regions of conglutinin contains three C-type lectin domains which can bind to carbohydrate structure on the α'-chain of iC3b as well as directly to carbohydrate structures on yeast, bacteria, and viruses. The human equivalent form has not been identified. The electron micrograph is from ref. 116.

C1s$_2$, is the physiologically more relevant protease with respect to the 'lectin route' of activation of the classical pathway (see *Figure 1.1*). It is not yet known if MASP is found as a dimer, or tetramer, or if it binds to MBP via the collagen-like regions of the molecule. After interaction of the C-type lectin modules present in the globular 'heads' of MBP, with carbohydrate structures present on yeasts, bacteria, and viruses, the MBP can mimic the action of C1q by activating MASP, or the $C1r_2$–$C1s_2$ complex, which in turn leads to the splitting of C4 and C2. It is considered that the C-type lectin module of MBP plays primarily a recognition role and that the collagen-like regions of the molecule interact with pro-enzyme MASP (or pro-enzyme $C1r_2$–$C1s_2$ complex) and also with the C1q receptor (after removal of the MASP or $C1r_2$–$C1s_2$ complex). The C-type lectin module of MBP contains approximately 130 residues of which 14 are invariant and 18 are highly conserved in character when compared with other C-type lectin modules showing different carbohydrate specificities (2). The C-type lectin domain of human MBP shows preferential binding to non-reducing, terminal, mannose, fucose, or glucosamine moieties in oligosaccharides. Despite the high conservation of the C-type lectin 'framework' of amino acid residues seen in MBP, conglutinin, and the lung surfactants SP-A and SP-D, these lectins show a remarkable divergence in selectivity of their carbohydrate binding properties with each lectin showing preferential binding to a distinct and different spectrum of sugars. This observation is consistent with the lectins' proposed function as innate antimicrobial agents. The three-dimensional structure of the MBP lectin module has been determined and is $40 \times 25 \times 25$ Å with more than half the structure in the form of loops and extended regions which are important in determining the, Ca^{2+}-dependent, carbohydrate-binding specificity of MBP. The remainder of the molecule is composed of a compact scaffold of two α helices and two β-sheets (6).

Conglutinin is a tetramer and, like MBP, its monomeric subunit is composed of three identical chains (2). Conglutinin is a more extended molecule due to the presence of a much larger stretch of collagen-like sequence in its unit polypeptide. Like MBP, each 'globular head' is composed of the three identical C-type lectin modules (*Figure 3.2b*).

Conglutinin binds to the single high-mannose oligosaccharide structures on the α' chain of iC3b as well as directly to carbohydrate structures on yeast, bacteria, and viruses. The binding of conglutinin to iC3b-coated Gram-negative bacteria enhances their killing by spleen and peritoneal exudate cells probably by mediating the binding of the iC3b-coated bacteria to the collectin/C1q receptor on phagocytes via the collagen-like region present in conglutinin.

2. The serine proteases of the complement system

All enzymes participating in the major steps concerned with activation (C1r, C1s, MASP, C2, factor B, factor D) and control (factor I) of the complement pathway belong to the family of mammalian serine proteases which include the digestive enzymes such as chymotrypsin and trypsin. The serine protease 'domain' has a M_r of approximately 23 000 Da with a characteristic 'triad' of active site residues His-57, Asp-102, Ser-195 (chymotrypsin numbering) comprising the charge relay system (7). (An exception is found in the anaphylatoxin inactivator, carboxypeptidase N, which removes the C-terminal Arg from C3a, C4a, and C5a.)

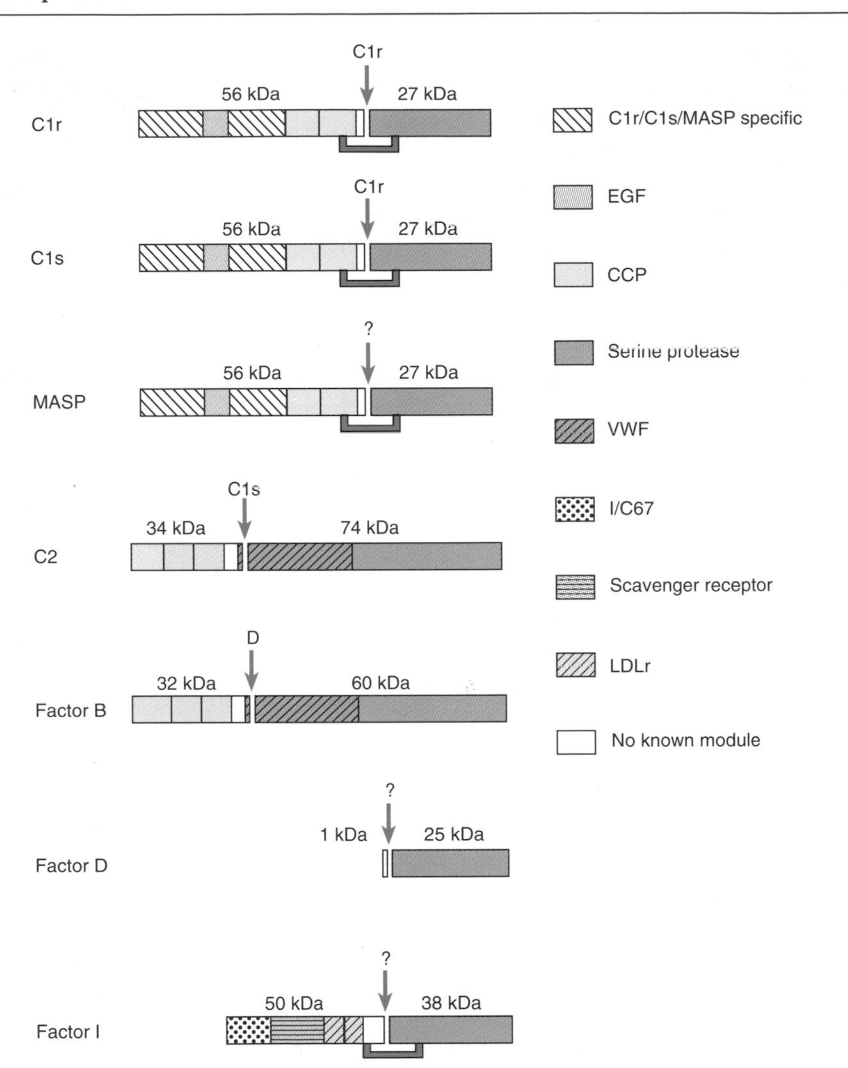

Figure 3.3. The serine proteases involved in the activation and control of the complement system. In addition to the serine protease domain, each of the proteins, except for factor D, has a large N-terminal portion composed of a collection of modular building blocks including the complement control protein (CCP) modules, epidermal growth factor (EGF) modules, von Willebrand factor (VWF) modules, low density lipoprotein receptor (LDLr) modules, scavenger receptor (SCr) modules, as well as the C1r/C1s-specific module which has only been identified in C1r, C1s, and MASP, and the (I/C67) module which has only been identified in factor I and the terminal components C6 and C7 (see *Figure 3.9*). The cleavage sites for activation of the components are marked and the disulphide bonds holding the cleaved polypeptides are shown in orange.

The complement serine proteases (and many of those in another cascade system—the blood clotting system), differ from the broadly specific, digestive enzymes (such as trypsin and chymostrypsin) by having a large polypeptide chain attached to the N-terminal of the serine protease domain (*Figure 3.3*). These fragments are thought to be involved in recognition and binding to suitable substrates and in limiting the protease activity to one or two bonds of the specific substrate molecules. It should be stressed that in most cases, a cofactor is also required. C1r, C1s, MASP, C2, and factor B circulate in the blood in their pro-enzyme forms. In contrast, only the activated forms of factor D and factor I have been found in circulation. Their respective pro-enzyme forms have not been isolated from plasma or serum samples, even after the addition of a wide spectrum of protease inhibitors. For the same reason, the proteases responsible for the conversion of the pro-enzyme forms to the active forms of factors D and I have not been identified.

2.1 C1r and C1s

C1r (8, 9) and C1s (10) are closely related proteins. They have a similar overall organization and when aligned, their primary sequences show about 40% identity. The genes encoding them have been located to chromosome 12 (p13) and the two genes are estimated to be only 20 kb apart in a tail-to-tail orientation (11). They are activated in a similar fashion. The native molecule, consisting of a single polypeptide, is cleaved into an N-terminal A-fragment of about M_r 56 000 Da and a C-terminal B-fragment of about M_r 27 000 Da joined by a single disulphide bond. Activation of C1r takes place when the C1 complex, via the C1q heads, binds to immune aggregates. A conformational change in the C1q complex takes place to allow the two C1r molecules to cleave, and activate, each other. The activated C1r, in turn, cleaves and activates C1s. The A-fragments of $C\overline{1r}$ and $C\overline{1s}$ contain three different types of repeating sequences (*Figure 3.3*). Two repeating sequences, occupying approximately residues 10–80 and 185–225, are present in both molecules. As similar sequences had not been identified in other proteins, they were called C1r/C1s-specific domains. It has recently been shown that the C1r/C1s module is present in MASP(5) and in a wide variety of vertebrate and invertebrate proteins, which are involved in developmental processes. An epidermal growth factor (EGF) module is found between the two C1r/C1s-specific domains and two complement control protein (CCP) domains are found at the C-terminal of the A-fragment. Although it is reasonable to propose that these 'extra' domains must play a regulatory role in delimiting the proteolytic activity of the serine protease domains of C1r and C1s to the few specific bonds of their respective substrates, the exact roles played by the various domains in the A-fragment can only be speculated. The EGF-like domain is relatively widespread in other protein families and may be involved in the self-association of the C1r and C1s in the Ca^{2+}-dependent C1s–C1r–C1r–C1s tetrameric complex, especially in view of the presence of β-hydroxylasparagine, which is known to bind Ca^{2+}, in these domains (12). The CCP repeats are the major building blocks of the regulatory proteins of complement activation (see Section 5) which bind activated fragments of C3 and C4. It is therefore reasonable to postulate that the two CCP repeats in C1r and C1s may be involved in binding C4 prior to its cleavage by $C\overline{1s}$.

2.2 Mannan-binding-protein-associated serine protease (MASP)

MASP (5) is present in serum in its pro-enzyme form as a chain of M_r 94 000 Da. Together MBP and MASP form what was previously described as Ra-reactive factor (RaRF) which is a serum bactericidal factor which activates C4 and C2 after binding to the Ra and R2 core polysaccharides found on many strains of enterobacteria such as *Salmonella* and *E. coli*. The MASP pro-enzyme, after activation, is composed of two chains, an N-terminal heavy chain of M_r 64 000 Da linked to a C-terminal light chain of M_r 30 000 Da. The light chain contains the serine protease domain. The heavy chain has the same domain structure as C1r and C1s, being composed of three module types, i.e. two of the 'C1r/C1s-specific' type, separated by an EGF module at the N-terminal end, followed by two CCP domains at the C-terminal end (*Figure 3.3*). The overall identity in amino acid sequence between MASP and C1r, or C1s, is approximately 37% (5).

2.3 Factor D

Factor D (13) has only been detected in its active form in plasma and serum samples as a single-chain protein of about M_r 25 000 Da. On comparison of the factor D sequence, obtained by protein sequencing, and the sequence derived from the cDNA clone of adipsin (13), the two proteins showed over 98% identity suggesting that they are in fact the same protein. (The minor differences are likely to be due to the incorrect assignment of residues at the protein level.) Thus, factor D/adipsin, in addition to its role in complement activation, may also play an essential role in lipid metabolism in adipose tissues. Unlike other serine proteases in the complement system, factor D does not have an N-terminal domain. Although the pro-D has not been detected in bodily fluids, it has been purified from culture medium of cells transfected with a cDNA clone. Two forms of pro-D molecule have been characterized, each with an activation peptide of either six (APPRGR) or seven (AAPPRGR) residues N-terminal to the serum form of factor D. Conversion of pro-D to factor D can be achieved by treatment with trypsin in laboratory conditions, but the natural activator of pro-D to factor D has not been identified (14).

In the complement system, there is only one known substrate of factor D, which is factor B, and the conversion of factor B to Ba and Bb requires the association of factor B with C3b or its equivalent form C3i. Recently, the three-dimensional structure of factor D has been determined by X-ray crystallography. The active site triad, i.e. the Asp-His-Ser triad, found in all serine proteases, is out of alignment and may therefore account for the absence of protease activity of factor D when examined on its own. It is possible that for activation, factor

D may require an induced-fit conformational change upon binding to factor B, which may provide the explanation for the very limited spectrum of substrates that can be cleaved by factor D (15).

2.4 Factor B and C2

The genes for factor B (6 kb) (16) and C2 (18 kb) (17) are located in the major histocompatibility complex (MHC) (see Section 3). The two proteins are similar to each other with over 40% identity in their amino acid sequences. The CCP repeats were first characterized in factor B (18) but were soon found to be the dominant structural element in the complement control proteins. Three CCP repeats are found in the N-terminal ends of factor B and C2. Activation of the two proteins, by factor D and the activated C1 complex respectively, involves the cleavage of a peptide bond C-terminal to the CCP repeats, giving N-terminal fragments of M_r 32 000 and M_r 34 000 Da in factor B and C2 respectively. For historical reasons, the N-terminal fragment in factor B is called Ba whereas that in C2 is called C2b. The larger C-terminal fragments are called Bb and C2a respectively and they both have a von Willebrand factor domain located N-terminal to the serine protease domain. Recent experiments suggest that the von Willebrand factor domain in factor B contains a binding site for C3b (19). It is interesting to note that a similar domain found on the complement receptor type 3 (CR3) has been shown to have iC3b binding activity (20).

2.5 Factor I

Factor I (21) is synthesized as a single chain precursor of M_r 88 000 Da which is processed to yield the active form, composed of two disulphide-linked chains (M_r 50 000 and 38 000 Da respectively), found in plasma. Although factor I is resistant to one of the classical serine protease inhibitors (i.e. diisopropyl-phosphofluoridate) the amino acid sequence of the light chain clearly shows that it is a member of the serine protease family. The heavy chain, which is the N-terminal fragment of the single chain precursor, is composed of four recognizable modular domains. They include, from the N-terminal, an I/C67-specific domain, a scavenger receptor domain, and two low density lipoprotein receptor (LDLr) domains. The I/C67-specific domain has only been found in factor I and in the terminal components C6 and C7. The scavenger receptor (SCr) domain has been identified in a number of cell-surface molecules including the CD5 and CD6 antigens, the scavenger receptor, the chemotactic receptor for the speract peptide in sea urchin, as well as a number of surface antigens of unknown function (22). The LDLr modules, first identified in the LDL receptor, have been found to distribute widely among many proteins including the components of the membrane attack complex of complement (see Section 7).

Factor I is not known to cleave proteins other than the complement components C3b and C4b and it can only do so in the presence of appropriate cofactors: factor H for C3b, C4bp for C4b, and CR1 and MCP for both (see *Table 2.1*).

3. Complement genes in the class III region of the major histocompatability complex (MHC)

The MHC is the name given to the genomic region where the antigens for transplantation compatability are coded. In man, it is located in chromosome 6 band p21.3 spanning a region of 3.5 mb (*Figure 3.4a*) (23). The MHC is divided into three regions. The genes encoding for the heavy chains of the class I antigen lie in the proximal 1.5 mb which is suitably called the class I region of the MHC. The heavy chain, together with the soluble β_2-microglobulin (coded for by a single gene in chromosome 15), form the class I antigens, which are expressed on all nucleated cells. The class II antigens are complexes of two membrane-bound polypeptides α and β, both encoded for by genes in the class II region, which occupies the distal 1.0 mb of the MHC. The class II antigens are restricted in their expression and are found only on cells and tissues involved in the regulation of T-cell differentiation. Both class I and class II antigens have similar structures, with a groove flanked by two α helices. Peptides are fitted in the grooves and are 'presented' to the T-cell receptor of cytotoxic (via class I antigens) or helper (via class II antigens) T cells. These interactions are extremely important in T-cell recognition and the regulation of both the cellular (T cells) and humoral (antibody production by B cells) immune responses (24). Antigen presentation not only involves the expression of the class I and class II antigens, but also the generation of peptides from foreign and self proteins and their transportation to the appropriate cellular compartment where they are incorporated into the class I and class II antigens before the complexes are expressed on the cell surface. It is therefore not surprising that genes encoding proteins for peptide transportation and intracellular proteolysis, among others, have recently been found in the class II region (25).

The region between class I and class II is called class III which spans approximately 1.0 mb of DNA. The first genes characterized in this region were the complement proteins C4, factor B, and C2 (26). Because of the polymorphism at the protein level, especially for C4, and the ease of obtaining samples from blood, these proteins were soon established as standard markers for MHC haplotyping. This became more important when it was found that certain diseases may correlate with the MHC haplotype of the patients (27). Since most of these diseases have a component of autoimmune irregularity, it was thought that certain polymorphic genes in this region, coding for products of the immune system, are responsible for the diseases. Clearly, the most logical candidates were the class I and class II antigens and C4. However, these correlations are not always clear cut and it was postulated that other polymorphic genes coding for proteins of the immune system would be found in this region. Systematic searching has yielded no less than 35 genes to date (25), but they are found to code for a diverse group of proteins with no obvious functional relationships. In view of the current understanding of antigen presentation, the correlation of autoimmune diseases with MHC haplotypes may not be directed to molecules of the immune system, but to peptides derived from a wide range of proteins

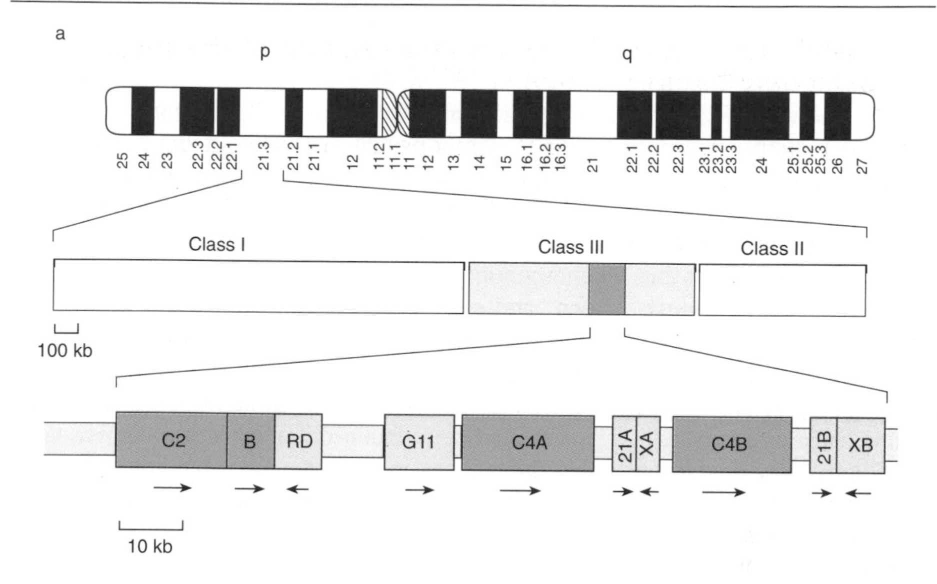

b

C4 Haplotypes	C4 Isotype expressed	Approximate frequency
A – B	A + B	70%
AQØ – B	B only	18%
B – B		
A – BQØ	A only	10%
A – A		
AQØ – BQØ	None	Very rare
A – A – B	A + B	1%
A – B – B		
A – B – B – B	A + B	One case

Figure 3.4. Complement genes in the major histocompatibility complex (MHC). (**a**) The location of the MHC in chromosome 6, band p21.3 covering approximately 3.5 mb. The complement genes and other genes found in the cluster are shown with the direction of the genes indicated. The C4 duplication unit includes the C4/CYP21/X genes. The CYP21A and XA in association with C4A are pseudogenes whereas the CYP21B gene codes for the adrenal steroid 21-hydroxylase and XB for a tenascin-like molecule (117). (Adapted from refs 23 and 25.) (**b**) Polymorphism of C4 gene expression. Genes in the C4A locus are in orange and genes in the C4B locus are grey. The nature of the locus is characterized by their similarity to the 'normal' C4A/C4B haplotype. However, the protein encoded, indicated by the letters A or B, may or may not match the locus type. Thus we have B-type locus expressing the C4A protein and *vice versa*. The genes in the QØ loci are not expressed. The haplotype frequencies are typical for Caucasoid populations (adapted from ref. 118.)

that play no active part in the immune system but are presented by the MHC class I and class II antigens.

Also shown in *Figure 3.4a* is a typical map of the region containing the genes of the complement proteins. This is only a partial map since it only represents 70% of the haplotypes found, and does not include others containing different numbers of C4 genes (*Figure 3.4b*). About 10% of the haplotypes have only one C4 gene in this region and one case having four C4 genes has been reported. It should be noted that this phenomenon is by no means unique to man. Some animals, including mouse, sheep, and cattle, also have multiple C4 genes, but others, including dog, cat, and guinea pig, appear to have only one copy (28). There are two types of C4 genes coding for the two C4 isotypes, C4A and C4B. Both C4A and C4B function effectively as C4 in the complement system. This is not surprising since their amino acid sequences differ by less than 1% (29). However, they have measurable differences in their covalent binding activities. C4A has very low binding activity to hydroxyl-group-containing compounds but is more effective in binding to amino-group containing compounds than C4B. C4B, on the other hand, binds to both hydroxyl and amino groups with similar efficiency (see Section 4). This is reflected in the more effective binding of C4B on erythrocyte surfaces, which are covered with hydroxyl groups on the carbohydrates of glycoproteins and glycolipids, which explains the higher specific haemolytic activity of C4B. On the other hand, C4A appears to bind more effectively to immune complexes, which are more proteinaceous in nature. Generally, C4A and C4B also differ in their antigenicity, with C4A carrying the Rodgers antigen and C4B the Chido antigen, as well as in their electrophoretic mobility, with C4A being more anionic. However, this generalization breaks down when examined at the allotypic level (30).

Perhaps because of the close proximity of the two genes and their extreme similarity, exchange of genetic information is frequent, leading to an array of C4 molecules with overlapping properties. To date, there have been about 35 allotypes of C4 described (31) and the most common ones and their properties are shown in *Figure 3.5*. Genetic variation is also evident at the genomic level including the number of C4 genes, C4B genes found in the C4A loci and *vice versa*, and genes not expressing a product. These variations can be detected by RFLP (restriction fragment length polymorphism) and other molecular biological techniques such as PCR (polymerase chain reaction). Typing can therefore be carried out at a higher resolution since it is not limited to the coding regions of functional genes.

The C4A6 allotype is unique in that it has very low, if detectable, haemolytic activity. It resembles other C4A allotypes in all respects except for its inability to form an active C5-convertase (32). The C4b–C3b covalent complex, the cofactor component of the C5-convertase (see Chapter 2, Section 4), has low affinity for C5 when formed with C4A6 (33). Sequencing at the DNA level shows an Arg to Trp substitution in the β-chain of C4A6, thus pinpointing the location of the C5 binding site on C4 (34,35). This finding also provides an explanation for C4A6 being the most anionic C4 allotype.

	C4A					C4B				
ALLOTYPE	A6	A4	A3	A2	A1	B5	B4	B3	B2	B1
Haemolytic activity	VL	L	L	L	L	H	H	H	H	H
Binding to $-NH_2$	+ + +	+ + +	+ + +	+ + +	+ + +	+	+	+	+	+
Binding to $-OH$	±	±	±	±	±	+	+	+	+	+
Antigenicity	Rg	Rg	Rg	Rg	Ch	Rg	Ch	Ch	Ch	Ch

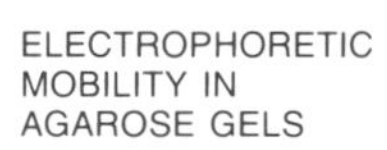

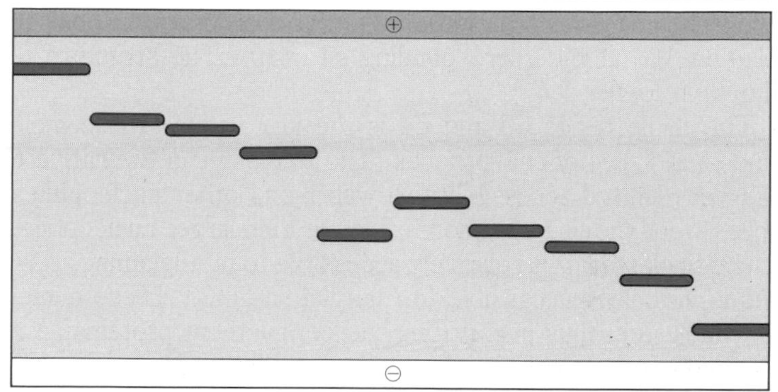

Figure 3.5. Properties of common C4 allotypes. Haemolytic activity: H = high, L = low, VL = very low. Reactivity of binding to amino and hydroxyl groups is indicated between highly reactive (+++) and marginally reactive (+/−). Antigenicity: Rg = Rodgers, Ch = Chido. It should be noted that all C4A allotypes have the sequence PCPVLD from position 1101 to 1106 and the C4B allotypes LSPVIH. Other variations in properties are due to residues outside this region (29,30).

Factor B and C2 are similar molecules, sharing 42% identity. The exonic organization of their genes are also similar (16). However, the overall size of the two genes differ remarkably, with factor B gene about 6 kb and C2 gene 18 kb. The difference is not due to the insertion/deletion of a single stretch of DNA, but to the generally larger introns in C2. This is particularly interesting since the C4 genes have a relatively uniform length of 16 or 22 kb. The difference lies in the presence of a single insertion of 6 kb in one of the introns of all C4A genes and some of the C4B genes. In addition, the factor B and C2 genes are about 500 bp apart and some of the regulatory elements of the factor B gene are found within the 3′ exons of the C2 gene (36).

4. C3, C4, and C5

C3 (37), C4 (38, 39), and C5 (40) are synthesized as single polypeptides which are subsequently processed into the multi-chain structures. An internal tetrapeptide of basic residues is removed from the pro-C3 and pro-C5 molecules yielding an N-terminal β chain and a C-terminal α chain covalently linked by disulphide bonds. A similar tetratpeptide is removed at the β–α junction of pro-C4. In addition, a stretch of 26 residues inclusive of four arginine residues at the C-terminal end is also removed at the α–γ junction. The three chains in C4 are also disulphide linked. C3 and C4 each have an internal thiolester which is formed between the Cys and the Gln residues of the tetrapeptide sequence of -Cys-Gly-Glu-Gln- found in their respective α chains (41). This thiolester is also found in the serum protease inhibitor α_2-macroglobulin (α_2M) and its related molecules, including the pregnancy zone protein (42). C5, which does not have the internal thiolester and does not bind covalently to cell surfaces, has the sequence -Ser-Ala-Glu-Ala- at the corresponding site (40). The structure of the thiolester is shown in *Figure 3.6.*

The thiolester in C3 and C4 is the key to how these molecules are able to bind to all types of cell surfaces. The thiolester in the native C3 and C4 protein has very limited accessibility to water and other nucleophiles. Smaller nucleophiles were shown to be more effective than larger nucleophiles in gaining access to the thiolester: it is relatively accessible to methylamine, less so to ethylamine, and is virtually inaccessible to *t*-butylamine (43). These nucleophiles react with the thiolester, thus inactivating the complement proteins. Activation of C3 and C4 involves the cleavage of a single peptide bond resulting in the dissociation of C3a and C4a, which constitute the first 77 amino acids of the α chains of C3 and C4, respectively, from the major fragments of C3b and C4b. This induces a gross conformational change of C3b and C4b which may be considered, in effect, as exposing the thiolester to allow it to react with water and other nucleophiles. On surfaces where complement is activated, the most common nucleophiles are hydroxyl groups on carbohydrates and amino groups on proteins. A fraction, in the order of 10%, of the C3b and C4b activated, would react with the surface hydroxyl and amino groups to become covalently bound to the surface via ester

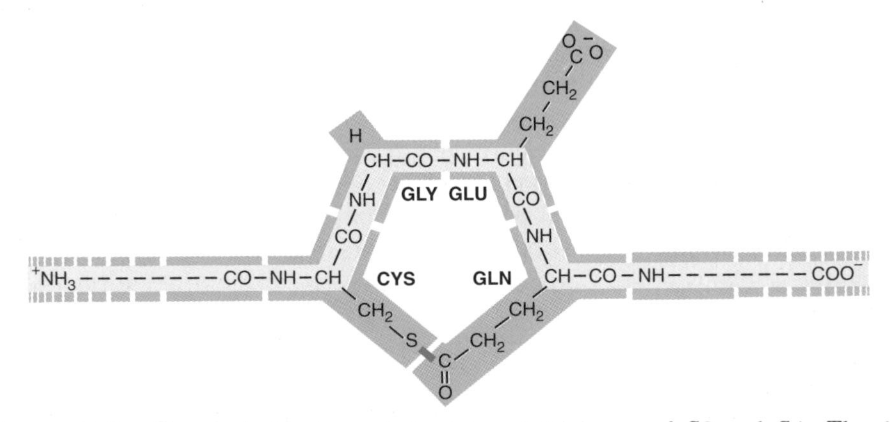

Figure 3.6. Chemical structure of the internal thiolester of C3 and C4. The 15-membered thiolactone ring is formed form four amino acid residues (on orange background), with a thiolester bond (orange) between Cys and Gln. The peptide backbone is indicated by the grey line. The structure is conserved in most C3, C4, and α_2-macroglobulin molecules except that Gly may be substituted by an Ala in some cases.

and amide bonds. It is thus rationalized that by reacting with the most common chemical groups, C3b and C4b can be deposited on all cell surfaces and serve as universal opsonins without any specificity at the biological level. Interestingly, C3, the two isotypes of C4, C4A and C4B, and α_2M react differently with amino and hydroxyl groups (44) (*Table 3.1*). Since C4A and C4B differ only by four amino acid residues in their primary structure, it is reasonable to assume that these four residues play a part in conferring binding specificity. Using site-directed mutagenesis at the cDNA level, these residues have been modified one at a time in a C4 cDNA, and the binding properties of the expressed proteins were found to correlate with the residue at position 1106. If the residue is a His, then the protein behaves like C4B. If the residue is an Asp, Ala, or Asn, then the protein is C4A-like (45, 46). Based on these observations, it was argued that the His in C4B is responsible for catalysing the reaction of the thiolester with

Table 3.1 The reaction of the thiolester in C3 and C4 with amino and hydroxyl groups (adapted from refs 44 and 46)

		Reaction rate k'/k_0 (M^{-1})[b]	
Proteins	Residues[a] 1101–1106	Glycine (amino group)	Glycerol (hydroxyl group)
Plasma proteins			
Human C3	DAPVI**H**	0	23.0
Human C4A	PCPVL**D**	13 400	1.3
Human C4B	LSPVI**H**	120	15.5
Human α_2M	SGSLL**N**	206	1.2
Mouse C4	PCPVI**H**	136	25.0
Modified human C4 (expressed proteins from cell culture)[c]			
Human C4-3	DAPVI**H**	125	14.0
Human C4-m	PCPVL**D**	210	16.0
Human C4-AA	PCPVL**A**	20 000	3.4
Human C4-BA	LSPVI**A**	22 000	3.2
Human C4-α	SGSLL**N**	15 000	1.0

[a] The residues 1101 to 1106 are the only different ones found between the human C4A and C4B isotypes and they may be referred to as the isotypic residues. The equivalent residues of C3, α_2M, and mouse C4 are obtained by alignment of the primary sequence of the proteins. In bold are residues at position 1106 which controls the reaction of the thiolester with amino and hydroxyl groups.

[b] The binding to glycine and glycerol depends on the reaction rate of the thiolester and the concentration of the small molecules. If the hydrolysis rate of the thiolester is k_0, and the reaction rate with glycine or glycerol is k', then the ratio of the protein bound with glycine or glycerol is given by $k'[G]/(k_0 + k'[G])$. This value can be determined experimentally by activating the thiolester proteins in the presence of known concentrations of radiolabelled glycine or glycerol. The value of k'/k_0 can be calculated accordingly.

[c] A human cDNA clone was modified to contain sequences encoding residues 1101 to 1106 from different origins. The resultant clones were C4-3 (residues from human C3), C4-m (mouse C4), C4-α (human α_2M), C4-AA (human C4A except for an alanine at position 1106), and C4-BA (human C4B except for an alanine at position 1106). The modified clones were transfected into an expression system and the proteins obtained were studied for their binding activities. These proteins differ from each other only at the positions shown.

hydroxyl groups, including water. In the absence of the His, this reaction is not catalysed and the reaction of the thiolester with the more nucleophilic amino groups would apparently become more dominant. This interpretation led to the prediction that the thiolester in C4A, upon activation, would be more stable to hydrolysis than that in C4B. Indeed, it was found that the half-life of activated C4A is over ten seconds, whereas that of activated C4B is less than one second (46).

This also provides an explanation of the presence of C4A and C4B in mammals. C4B has been found in all mammals studied and may be presumed to be more important. This view is emphasized by the finding that only in animals with more than one C4 gene can one find C4A genes (28). Thus, it may be interpreted that only the animals with 'spare' copies of the C4B genes can have the propensity to convert one of their genes to code for a C4A-like product. Since there is no specific residue that confers a C4A-like activity, C4A may be regarded as C4B having lost its catalytic capability of reacting with hydroxyl groups and water at the thiolester site.

Whether C4A is important in our health is open to debate. Deficiency in C4A, both in heterozygous and homozygous states, correlates with the incidence of autoimmune disorders such as systemic lupus erythematosus (SLE) (47), suggesting that it may play a morc important role than C4B in the clearance of immune complexes. C4A may also be important in the induction of the immune response. Guinea pigs genetically deficient in C4 have a subnormal antibody response, both in the primary and secondary responses, when immunized with the bacteriophage $\phi\chi$ 174. If purified human C4A, or guinea pig C4, but not human C4B, is included in the primary injection of the immunogen, both the primary and secondary responses to $\phi\chi$ 174 appear normal (48). However, this interpretation does not appear to be consistent with the finding that normal guinea pig serum has only one C4 protein which is C4B-like in character (28).

The genes coding for C3, C4, C5, and α_2M are not linked. In man, they are located on different chromosomes: C3 in chromosome 19, C4 in chromosome 6, C5 in chromosome 2, and α_2M in chromosome 12. These four proteins are found to be similar to each other throughout the entire coding sequence and the exonic organization of their genes is also similar. It is therefore likely that they are evolved from a common ancestral gene. These proteins belong to a closed family in that no region within these proteins is found in any protein outside this family. The higher order structure of the thiolester proteins is not known.

5. Regulators of complement activation (RCA) and related proteins

It was first observed in the primary structure of factor B that there are three repeating elements at the N-terminal end. Each repeating element is encoded by a single exon in the factor B gene (18). Similar structural motifs were soon found in other complement proteins (*Figure 3.7*). Of particular interest are the proteins that regulate C3 and C4 activation and degradation: (i) they are composed predominantly of these repeating structures, and (ii) their genes are located in a cluster, called the RCA (regulator of complement activation) gene cluster, in chromosome 1 band q32 of man. These proteins include soluble proteins factor H and the α and β subunits of C4bp, and membrane proteins CR1, CR2, MCP, and DAF (49). The repeating elements have been referred to as SCRs (short consensus repeats) or more appropriately CCP (complement control protein) repeats.

Each CCP repeat is about 60 residues in length and is characterized by a framework of highly conserved residues including four Cys which were found to form two disulphide bonds in the 1–3 and 2–4 pattern. By two-dimensional NMR, the three-dimensional structures of several CCP repeats have been determined (50). The sequence and ribbon diagram of a representative CCP module (the 16th CCP module of factor H) are shown in *Figure 3.8*. CCP repeats are also found in factor B and C2 (genes in chromosome 6p 21.3), C1r and C1s (genes in chromosome 12 p13), and C6 and C7 (genes in chromosome 5q).

It should be stressed that CCP repeats are not found exclusively in complement proteins. At least one other protein, the β subunit of the blood clotting factor XIII, is coded by a gene within the RCA gene cluster (49). Other human proteins containing CCP repeats include the β_2-glycoprotein I, the interleukin-2 receptor, and the cartilage proteoglycan core protein. CCP repeats are also found in proteins very distant from man, for example in a serine protease inhibitor in *Limulus*, and in a vaccinia virus protein capable of regulating the activation of the human complement pathway (51).

A variant form of the CCP repeat has also been identified in the selectins (51). These variant repeats contain two additional cysteine residues. However, the sequences of these repeats can be fitted easily to the three-dimensional coordinates of the complement repeats with the two extra cysteines in close proximity and may be presumed to engage in a disulphide bond (50). The three selectin genes are found in a region encompassing 300 kb on chromosome 1q 21–24.

Higher order organization of the CCP repeats are found in human CR1 (52, 53) and CR2 (54, 55). Both are type I membrane proteins (i.e. with the N-terminal portion extracellular and separated from the C-terminal cytoplasmic end by a single stretch of about 25 hydrophobic residues). The extracellular portions of both CR1 and CR2 consist exclusively of CCP repeats. The most common allotypes (82%) of CR1 have 30 CCP repeats with the N-terminal 28 residues organized into four long homologous repeats (LHR), designated A, B, C, and D from the N-terminal, each containing seven CCP repeats (53). The corresponding CCP repeats in the LHRs are highly conserved with repeats 3 in LHR-B and LHR-C having identical sequences. Repeats 3–7 of LHR-A and LHR-B are over 99% identical and repeats 1–4 of LHR-B and LHR-C are over 95% identical. Discrete numbers of CCPs were removed at the cDNA level and the shortened CR1s were expressed and studied for their binding to C3b and C4b. It was determined that CR1 has one C4b binding site and two C3b binding sites. The

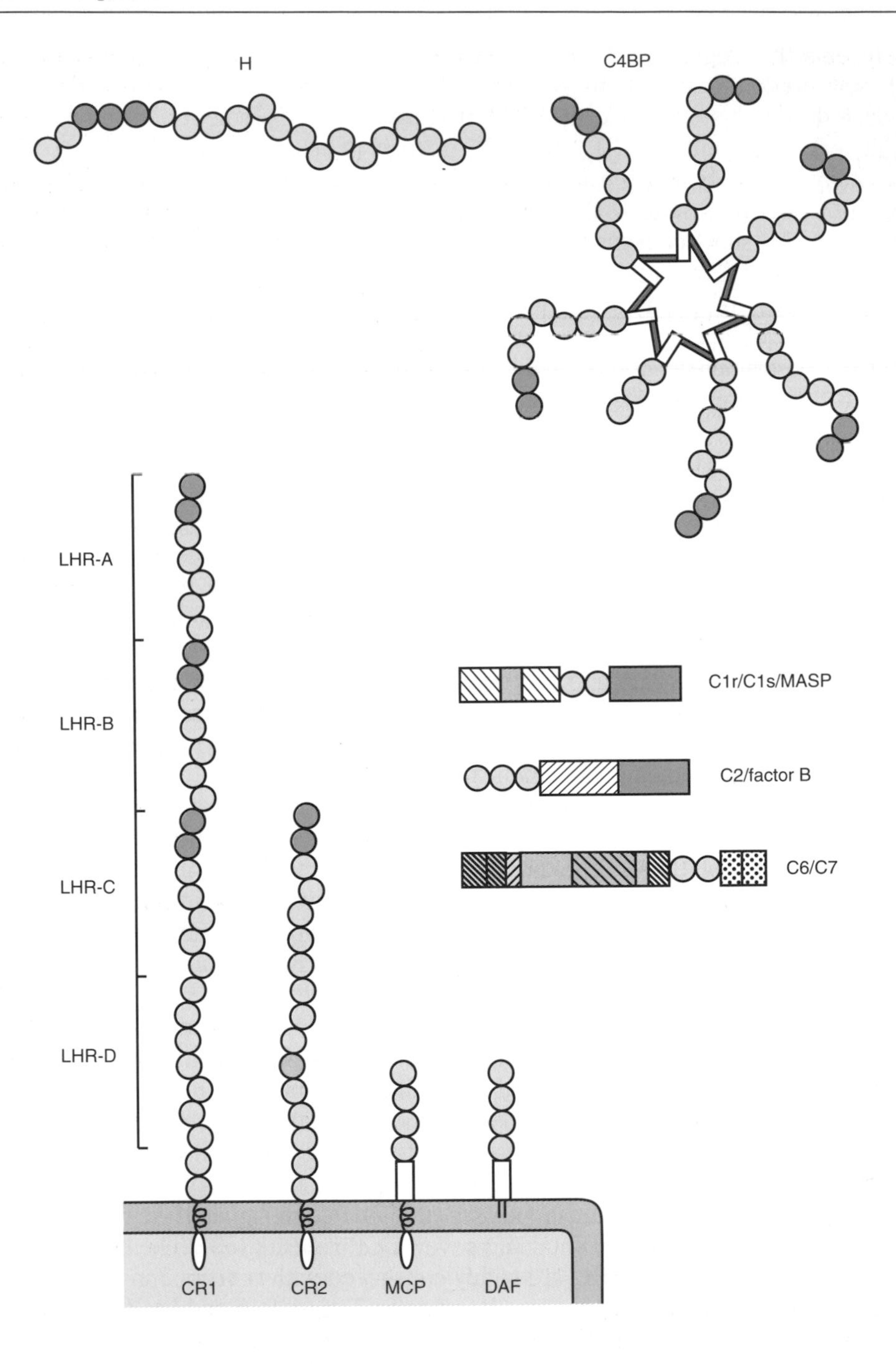
H
C4BP
LHR-A
LHR-B
LHR-C
LHR-D
C1r/C1s/MASP
C2/factor B
C6/C7
CR1
CR2
MCP
DAF

Figure 3.7. Regulators of complement activation (RCA). These proteins are coded in a gene cluster in chromosome 1 band q32. An outstanding feature is that they are composed predominantly of the complemenent control protein (CCP) repeats (also referred to as the short consensus repeats, SCR). Higher order structures are found with CR1. Shown in the figure is the most abundant allotype (82%) with four long homologous repeats (LHR) each containing seven CCPs. LHR-A contains a binding site for C4b and LHR-B and LHR-C binding sites for C3b. CCP units forming the binding sites for C3 or C4 fragments are in orange. The eleventh CCP repeat in CR2 (shaded in grey) may or may not be expressed depending on alternative splicing. DAF is membrane bound via a glycosyl phosphatidylinositol anchor. The 6α1β version of C4BP is shown with the interchain disulphide bonds in orange. Also shown are the other complement proteins containing CCP repeats: they are C1r, C1s, C2, factor B, C6, and C7. Other modules of these proteins can be found in *Figures 3.3* and *3.9*. Their genes are not located in the RCA cluster.

C4b binding site is located in LHR-A and the two C3b binding sites in LHR-B and LHR-C respectively. It has also been determined that the binding sites for C3b and C4b require the presence of at least the first three CCP repeats within the LHR. Thus, CR1 may be regarded as a composite receptor. The arrangement of binding sites on the same protein may provide multivalent interaction between CR1 and C3b and C4b on immune complexes, to facilitate their clearance. The next most frequent CR1 allotype (17%) has an additional LHR between LHR-A and LHR-B. This extra LHR, by primary sequence analysis, also appears to contain a C3b binding site (56).

Two forms of CR2 are expressed, containing 15 or 16 (extra one at 11) CCP repeats in the extracellular domain. Four long-range repeats can also be identified, each containing four CCP repeats in the 16 repeat version (57). The degree of similarity between the LHRs is not as striking as that for CR1. CR2 has a single binding site which recognizes iC3b, C3dg, and C3d. The binding site is located at the first two CCP repeats of CR2 (58).

DAF (59, 60) and MCP (61) each contain four CCP repeats at the N-terminal followed by a stretch of Ser/Thr-rich sequence where O-linked carbohydrates are found. DAF is anchored to the membrane by a GPI-anchor whereas MCP contains a classical hydrophobic segment of about 25 residues. The C3b/C4b binding sites are located within the region containing the CCP repeats. DAF and MCP are distributed widely in cells and tissues and are presumed to play a critical role in regulating C3 activation on host cells (62, 63).

C4bp has a very unusual structure. Seven polypeptides, each containing eight CCP repeats (64), are linked via disulphide bonds near the C-terminal to yield a 'spider-like' structure (65). Although previously thought to be composed of a single type of polypeptide (α chain), it has recently been shown that another polypeptide containing three CCP repeats (β chain) is occasionally found in the C4bp complex (66). Thus the complex could be of the composition of 7α0β or 6α1β. The α and β chains of C4bp are coded for by different genes, both of which are located in the RCA cluster (67). It has been shown that the first three

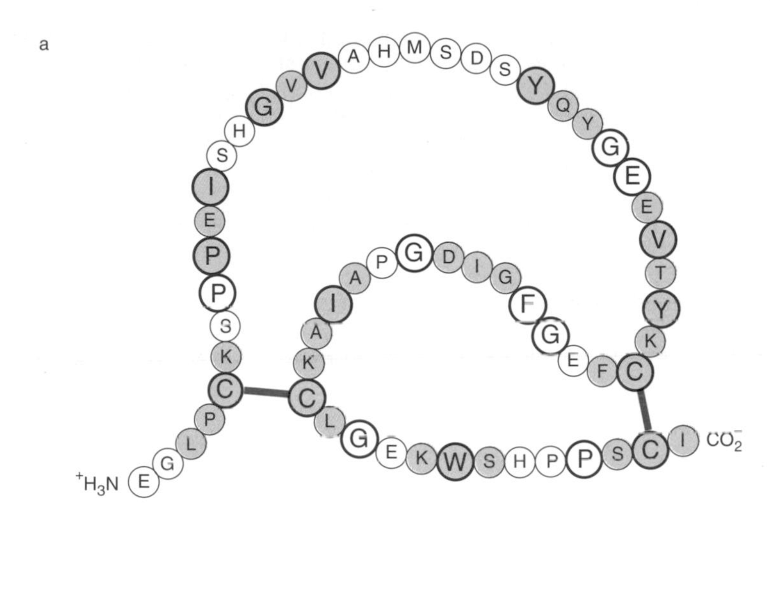

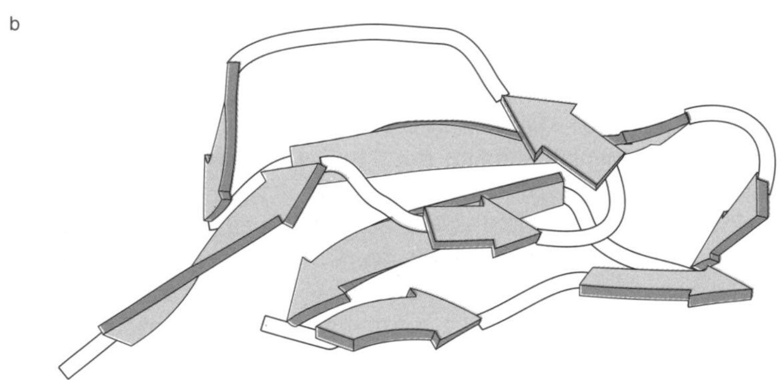

Figure 3.8. Complement control protein (CCP) module. (**a**) The sequence of the 16th CCP repeat of human factor H (H-16). The amino acids are in single letter code (see Abbreviations). Highly conserved residues in CCP modules are shown in bold. Shaded residues are located in the β-strands shown in (**b**). The two disulphide bonds between the two pairs of cysteines are shown in orange. (**b**) The ribbon diagram of the CCP module H-16 showing the a globular structure with a series of β-strands (broad arrows) connected with loops and turns. (Drawn by Dr A. J. Day based on two-dimensional NMR data from ref. 50.)

CCP repeats of the α chain contain the C4b binding site. It is not known if the β chain has C4b binding activity.

Factor H is composed exclusively of CCP repeats (68). The first five repeats have been shown to contain cofactor activity for fluid phase C3b (69). However, the regulation of factor H on surface-bound C3b may be more complex. For example, it is known that the presence of sialic acid on sheep erythrocytes promotes the binding of factor H on surface-bound C3b, thus sheep erythrocytes are not capable of activating the alternative pathway of human complement. Upon enzymatic removal of the sialic acid from the cell surface, factor H interacts less effectively with surface-bound C3b thus allowing the activation of the alternative pathway to take place (70). It was subsequently shown that factor H contains an additional binding site, distinct for the C3b binding site, for sialic acid and other polyanions (71).

Other factor-H-like molecules containing varying numbers of CCP repeats have been reported at the protein and cDNA level, some of which are alternatively spliced products of the factor H gene; others are likely to be products of factor-H-related genes (72, 73). The activities of these proteins, which may or may not be related to the complement system, have not been characterized.

6. Components of the membrane attack complex (MAC)

A striking feature of the terminal components of complement is the manner in which a group of soluble hydrophilic components (C5b, C6, C7, C8, and C9) rapidly undergo a hydrophilic–amphiphilic transition via a non-enzymatic, self-assembly mechanism to form the membrane attack complex (MAC) containing up to 18 molecules of C9, which behaves as an integral membrane protein complex.

The C6 (74, 75), C7 (76), C8α (77), C8β (78, 79), and C9 (80) components of the MAC are structurally and functionally related. Primary structure analysis has shown that this group of proteins is unusual in that they are composites of many different modules. A core structure, which is shared by all five proteins, consists of a thrombospondin (TSR) module, an LDLr module, a MAC-specific domain, a lytic domain, and an EGF-like module. Comparison of their amino acid sequences in this region shows 28–35% identity between any pair of sequences. This is also the complete structural organization of the C9 molecule. Other components have additional domains at the N- and C-terminals of this organization. C8α and C8β have an extra TSR module at the C-terminal. In addition to the TSR module, C6 and C7 have two CCP modules and two factor I/C67-specific modules C-terminal to the TSR module. Finally, an additional TSR module is found at the N-terminal end of C6.

The key domain in the MAC component is the lytic domain, which is also found in perforin (81), the lytic molecule released from intracellular granules by cytotoxic T cells upon activation. The lytic domain is about 200 residues in length and they are about 25% identical to each other. Perforin also has an EGF-like module C-terminal to the lytic domain. However, the two regions, one at the N-terminal and the other at the C-terminal of perforin, each of about 150 residues, show no similarity to the MAC components nor to any other known proteins (see *Figure 3.9*).

Perforin requires Ca^{2+}, but not other proteins, to generate lytic activity. The

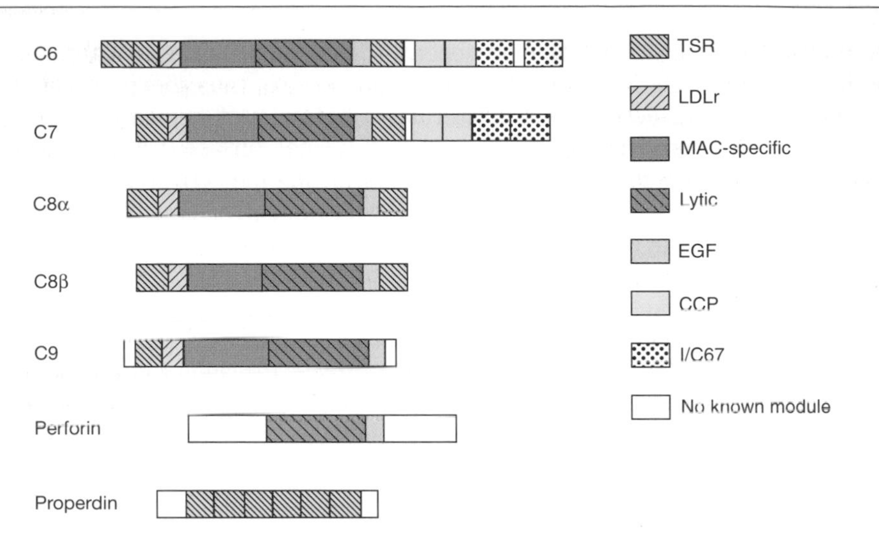

Figure 3.9. The modular structure of the complement MAC components and properdin. The common feature of the terminal complement components is the lytic domain which is also found in perforin, the T-cell cytotoxic molecule which lyses targets in a similar fashion to the complement proteins. Other modules include the thrombospondin (TSR) module, the LDLr module, the EGF module, CCP module, a module only found in factor I and C6 and C7 (I/C67) to date, and a region specific for the MAC components. The TSR module is also found in properdin, the six repeating units are flanked by short, highly charged regions at both the N- and C-termini.

cylindrical structures on the membrane of the perforin-lysed targets, as viewed by electron microscopy, have very similar appearance to those on MAC-lysed targets (81, 82). In this regard, under appropriate conditions (>40°C and under limited denaturing conditions), purified C9 can also polymerize to form the cylindrical structures (83). Under physiological conditions, however, the other four components, namely C6, C7, C8α, and C8β, in addition to C5b, are required for efficient cell lysis. It should be noted that C8γ (84), which is structurally unrelated to the other complement components, is not required for lytic activity. Its function in the complement system remains unknown.

The sequential assembly of C5 to C9 may provide multiple regulation points of the lytic activity of complement. For example, it is known that the C5b6 complex is more readily bound to cell surfaces coated with C3b. The binding of C7 to C5b6 forms the trimolecular C5b67 complex which either binds to the membrane of a target cell, or forms self-aggregates, or binds to inhibitory proteins in the fluid phase, such as the S-protein (vitronectin) and SP40,40. Membrane-bound C5b67 is stable and serves as a lytic site for the sequential incorporation of C8 via its β subunit, and C9, which binds to the α subunit of C8. The binding of the first molecule of C9 to C8 induces a conformational change in the molecule and initiates the polymerization of C9 to form the pore-like structures (85).

The mosaic structure of the terminal components remains an enigma. The core structures of the four proteins, C6, C7, C8α, and C8β, are similar to that of C9 but none of them can form the pore-like lesion on cell membranes. Although it is reasonable to speculate that these extra domains must serve some regulatory functions, exactly why they are distributed as such in the individual complement components remains unclear.

7. MAC inhibition factors

A set of unrelated proteins is known to inhibit the MAC lytic activity. After complement activation, MAC complexes can be found in the fluid phase as well as on target membrane. The MAC isolated from the fluid phase, when analysed, has been found to contain an additional protein which is called the S-protein. It binds to the complex at the stage of C5b67. Thus when the newly formed complex is not bound to the target membrane, the S-protein will irreversibly bind to the complex and abolish its membrane binding activity. The S-protein was subsequently purified and shown to be vitronectin (86). Vitronectin is a cell spreading factor present in plasma as well as on the surface of many cells, connective tissues, and platelets. It may serve as a local regulator of MAC formation on host cells during inflammatory conditions.

Another protein, SP40,40, has been shown to associate with the terminal complex in human glomerular immune deposits. It has complement inhibitory activity similar to the S-protein by binding to activated C5b67. SP40,40 is a soluble protein found in the blood at a level of 50 to 100 $\mu g\ ml^{-1}$. Sequence analysis shows that SP40,40 (87, 88) is highly homologous to the protein clusterin (also called SGP-2 for Sertoli cell glycoprotein-2) in the seminal fluid of the rat. Subsequently, the human form was detected in the seminal fluid of normal individuals at a range of 2 to 15 $mg\ ml^{-1}$. *In vitro* tests show a correlation between the fertility of semen samples and the concentration of SP40,40 (89). However, whether this correlation is due to the MAC inhibitory activity of SP40,40 is not known.

It has been a long-observed phenomenon that the lytic activity of MAC is significantly lower on cells from the same species. The presence of a membrane-bound inhibitor was postulated. Since the inhibitor acts in a species-specific manner, it was called the homologous restriction protein. In fact, two of these proteins had been found. One is CD59, which anchors to the membrane via a glycosyl phosphatidylinositol (GPI)-linker (90). It acts by inhibiting the polymerization of C9 on the C5b-8 complex, although it does not appear to interfere with the initial C9 binding to the α chain of C8 (91). Since it was characterized in several laboratories, it has been referred to variously as HRF20, MACIF, protectin, MIRL, and MEM-43-Ag. CD59 is also found in extracellular vesicles in seminal plasma and is proposed to have a protective function for spermatozoa against complement activities (92). Another membrane-bound MAC inhibitory protein of M_r ~60 000 Da has been reported as the homologous restriction factor (HRF), MIP, C8bp, and C9bp. It also appears to attach to the membrane via a

GPI-anchor and has a wide tissue distribution. However, its primary structure remains to be determined (93).

8. Properdin

Properdin (94) is present in plasma primarily in the form of dimers (P2), trimers (P3), and tetramers (P4) of a M_r 53 000 Da polypeptide chain. These oligomers have a very constant distribution of 26:25:20, for the P2:P3:P4 forms, respectively. The M_r 53 000 Da chain of properdin is composed of six tandemly repeating motifs, each of approximately 60 amino acids long, flanked by short, highly charged, N-terminal and C-terminal regions (*Figure 3.9*) (94). The formation of the oligomeric forms is considered to be due to strong ionic interactions between the N- and C-terminal ends of different chains (see *Figure 2.11*). The repeating motifs show a strong similarity to the type 1 repeats first described in the cell adhesion protein thrombospondin (95) and therefore the motif is usually known as the thrombospondin (TSR) module. Modules of this type are also seen in the terminal components of complement (*Figure 3.9*), the F-spondin protein, and also in certain parasite proteins, for example the circumsporozoite protein of the malaria parasite (96). In each case it is possible that the TSR modules play an adhesion role but this requires further work for clarification.

9. Complement receptors and the integrins

C3b in serum is rapidly converted to iC3b by factor I and its cofactors. Even on activating surfaces of the alternative pathway where this conversion is retarded, a substantial level of iC3b is found. However, the subsequent conversion of iC3b to C3c and C3dg by serum proteases is relatively slow. Hence the majority of bound C3 fragments on target surfaces is in the form of iC3b (97). It is therefore not surprising that a receptor specific to iC3b is required to partake in the elimination of opsonized targets. CR3 is found on phagocytes and its binding to iC3b requires divalent cations. In addition to ligand binding, CR3 appears to play an important role in the ingestion process (see Chapter 4, Section 4).

CR3 belongs to a group of adhesion molecules now commonly known as the integrins (98), which are characterized structurally by their αβ heterodimeric subunit composition and functionally by their interaction with multiple ligands in a divalent-cation-dependent fashion. CR3 is a member of the β2 subgroup (99) in which the β2 integrin subunit (100, 101) interacts with one of the three α subunits to form the three members of the leukocyte integrins. It combines with the αL subunit (102) to form the LFA-1 antigen (αLβ2), the αM subunit (103, 104, 105) to form CR3 or the Mac-1 antigen (αMβ2), and the αX subunit (106) to form the p150,95 antigen.

The three integrins bind to a variety of ligands and play important roles in many activities involving leukocyte adhesion (98, 107). Of particular interest is the binding of CR3 and p150,95, but not LFA-1, to iC3b. The role of CR3 in the phagocytosis of iC3b-coated targets has been well documented (108). The binding of p150,95 to iC3b-bearing cells is more difficult to assess since p150,95 is only expressed at low levels, in comparison to CR3, on cells easily available for experiments. Although the affinity of detergent-solubilized p150,95 for iC3b has been demonstrated at low ionic strengths (109, 110), its role as a complement receptor (CR4) has not been fully established.

The I domain is present in all three α subunits of the leukocyte integrins. This domain is found to be similar to a region first described for the von Willebrand factor. More importantly, in the context of complement, similar domains are found in C2 and factor B. It has been demonstrated that this domain in CR3 binds divalent cations and contains the binding site for iC3b (20). Similarly, the domain in factor B has been shown to have C3b binding activity (19).

iC3b is not the only ligand of CR3 (108). CR3 appears to have the capacity to bind to a wide range of ligand molecules including soluble proteins, such as the blood clotting factor X and fibrinogen, surface immobilized protein such as iC3b, authentic membrane proteins like ICAM-1, extracellular matrix proteins such as fibronectin, and other non-protein molecules such as bacterial lipopolysaccharide (LPS). Two non-overlapping sets of monoclonal antibodies have been shown to block either iC3b binding or LPS binding. Thus there are at least two distinct binding sites on CR3.

10. C5a receptor and G-protein complexes

The primary structure of the C5a receptor (111, 112) indicates that it is a member of the rhodopsin superfamily with a characteristic seven transmembrane helices. This finding is consistent with other biochemical evidence that the C5a receptor acts via a GTP-binding protein complex (113). The C5a receptor is closely related to the receptor for the bacterial chemotactic peptide *f*-Met-Leu-Phe (114) with about 35% sequence identity. This agrees with the suggestion that the two receptors mediate similar but not identical responses in neutrophils and monocytes.

11. Further reading

11.1 Molecular genetics of complement components

Dodds,A.W. and Day,A.J. (1993). In *Complement in health and disease* (ed. K.Whaley, M.Loos, and J.M. Weiler), p. 39. Immunology and Medicine Series 20. Kluwer Academic Publishers, London.

Reid,K.B.M. and Campbell,R.D. (1993). In *Complement in health and disease* (ed. K.Whaley, M.Loos, and J.M.Weiler), p. 89. Immunology and Medicine Series 20. Kluwer Academic Publishers, London.

11.2 C1q and related molecules

Behring Inst. Mitteilungen (1989). **84** (Entire volume).
Behring Inst. Mitteilungen (1993). **93** (Entire volume).
Holmskov,U. Malhotra,R., Sim,R.B., and Jensenius,J.C. (1994). *Immunol. Today*, **15,** 67.
Reid,K.B.M. (1983). *Biochem. Soc. Trans.*, **11,** 1.

11.3 MHC genetics and C4 polymorphism

Campbell,R.D. (1993). In *Genome analysis. Vol. 5: Regional physical mapping*, p. 1. Cold Spring Harbor Laboratory Press.
Kay,P.H. and Dawkins,R.L. (1987). In *Complement in health and disease* (ed. K.Whaley), p. 79. MTP, Lancaster.
Sim,E. and Dodds,A.W. (1987). In *Complement in health and disease* (ed. K.Whaley), p. 125. MTP, Lancaster.

11.4 Thiolester proteins

Sottrup-Jensen,L. (1987). In *The plasma proteins* (ed. F.W.Putnam), Vol. V, p.191. Academic Press, Florida.

11.5 MAC components and MAC inhibitors

Morgan,B.P. (1993). In *Complement in health and disease* (ed. K.Whaley, M.Loos, and J.M.Weiler), p. 325. Immunology and Medicine Series 20. Kluwer Academic Publishers, London.

11.6 Proteins of the RCA family

Hourcade,D., Holers,V.M., and Atkinson,J.P. (1989). *Adv. Immunol.*, **45,** 381.

11.7 C3 receptors

Ahearn,J.M. and Fearon,D.T. (1989). *Adv. Immunol.*, **46,** 183.
Hynes,R.O. (1993). *Cell*, **69,** 11.
Law,S.K.A. (1993). In *Blood cell biochemistry* (ed: M.A.Horton), Vol. 5, p. 223. Plenum, New York.

11.8 Chemotactic receptors

Gerard,C. and Gerard,N.P. (1994). *Curr. Opin. Immunol.*, 6, 140.

12. References

1. Reid,K.B.M. (1983). *Biochem. Soc. Trans.*, **11,** 1.
2. Holmskov,U., Malhotra,R., Sim,R.B., and Jensenius,J.C. (1994). *Immunol. Today*, **15,** 67.
3. Matsushita,M. and Fujita,T. (1992). *J.Exp.Med.*, **176,** 1497.
4. Ji,Y., Fujita,T., Hatsuse,H., Takahashi,A., Matsushita,M., and Kawakami,M. (1993). *J. Immunol.*, **150,** 571.
5. Takada,F., Takayama,Y., Hatsuse,H., and Kawakami,M. (1993). *Biochem. Biophys. Res. Commun.*, **196,** 1003.
6. Weis,W.I., Drickamer,K., and Hendrickson,W.A. (1992). *Nature*, **360,** 127.
7. Neurath,H. (1984). *Science*, **224,** 350.

8. Journet,A. and Tosi,M. (1986). *Biochem.J.*, **240,** 783.
9. Leytus,S.P., Kurachi,K., Sakariassen,K.S., and Davie,E.W. (1986). *Biochemistry*, **25,** 4855.
10. Tosi,M., Duponchel,C., Meo,T., and Julier,C. (1987). *Biochemistry*, **26,** 8516.
11. Kusumoto,H., Hirosawa,S., Salier,J.P., Hagen,F.S., and Kurachi,K. (1988). *Proc. Natl Acad. Sci. USA*, **85,** 7307.
12. Thielens,N.M., Van Dorsselaer,A., Gagnon,J., and Arlaud,G.J. (1990). *Biochemistry*, **29,** 3570.
13. White,R.T., Damm,D., Hancock,N., Rosen,B.S., Bradford,B.L., Usher,P., Flier,J.S., and Spiegelman,B.M. (1992). *J. Biol. Chem.*, **267,** 9210.
14. Yamauchi,Y., Stevens,J.W., Macon,K.J., and Volanakis,J.E. (1993). *Mol. Immunol.*, **30,** 63.
15. Narayana,S.V.L., Moore,D., DeLucas,L.J., Kilpatrick,J.M., Yamauchi,Y., Macon,K.J., and Volanakis,J.E. (1993). *Mol. Immunol.*, **30,** 37.
16. Campbell,R.D., Bentley,D.R., and Morley,B.J. (1984). *Phil. Trans. R. Soc. Lond. B*, **306,** 367.
17. Bentley,D.R. (1986). *Biochem. J.*, **239,** 339.
18. Morley,B.J. and Campbell,R.D. (1984). *EMBO J.*, **3,** 153.
19. Williams,S.C. and Sim,R.B. (1994). *Biochem. Soc. Trans.*, **22,** 2S.
20. Michishita,M., Videm,V., and Arnaout,M.A. (1993). *Cell*, **72,** 857.
21. Catterall,C.F., Lyons,A., Sim,R.B., Day,A.J., and Harris,T.J.R. (1987). *Biochem J.*, **242,** 849.
22. Law,S.K.A., Micklem,K.J., Shaw,J.M. Zhang,X.P., Dong,Y., Willis,A.C., and Mason,D.Y. (1993). *Eur. J. Immunol.*, **23,** 2320.
23. Campbell,R.D. (1993). In *Genome analysis.* Vol. 5: *Regional physical mapping*, p. 1. Cold Spring Harbor Laboratory Press.
24. Austyn,J.M. (1989). In *Antigen presenting cells* (ed. D.Male). In Focus Series. IRL, Oxford.
25. Campbell,R.D. and Trowsdale,J. (1993). *Immunol. Today*, **14,** 349.
26. Carroll,M.C., Campbell,R.D., Bentley,D.R., and Porter,R.R. (1984). *Nature*, **307,** 237.
27. Hansen,J.A. and Nelson,J.L. (1990). *CRC Crit. Rev. Immunol.*, **10**, 307.
28. Dodds,A.W. and Law,S.K.A. (1990). *Biochem. J.*, **265,** 495.
29. Yu,C.Y., Belt,K.T., Giles,C.M., Campbell,R.D., and Porter,R.R. (1986). *EMBO J.*, **5,** 2873.
30. Dodds,A.W., Law,S.K.A., and Porter,R.R. (1986). *Immunogenetics*, **24,** 279.
31. Mauff,G., Brenden,M., Braun-Stilwell,M., Doxiadis,G., Giles,C.M., Hauptmann,G., Rittner,C., Schneider,P.M., Stradmann-Bellinghausen,B., and Uring-Lambert,B. (1990). *Complement and Inflammation*, **7**, 193.
32. Dodds,A.W., Law,S.K.A., and Porter,R.R. (1985). *EMBO J.*, **4,** 2239.
33. Kinoshita,T., Dodds,A.W., Law,S.K.A., and Inoue,K. (1989). *Biochem. J.*, **261,** 743.
34. Anderson,M.J., Milner,C.M., Cotton,R.G.H., and Campbell,R.D. (1992). *J. Immunol.*, **148,** 2795.
35. Ebanks,R.O., Jaikaran,A.S.I., Carroll,M.C., Anderson,M.J., Campbell,R.D., and Isenman,D.E. (1992). *J. Immunol.*, **148,** 2803.
36. Wu,L.C., Morley,B.J., and Campbell,R.D. (1987). *Cell*, **48,** 331.
37. de Bruijn,M.H.L. and Fey,G.H. (1985). *Proc. Natl Acad. Sci. USA*, **82,** 708.
38. Belt,K.T., Carroll,M.C., and Porter,R.R. (1984). *Cell*, **36,** 907.
39. Belt,K.T., Yu,C.Y., Carroll,M.C., and Porter,R.R. (1985). *Immunogenetics*, **21,** 173.
40. Haviland,D.L., Haviland,J.C., Fleischer,D.T., Hunt,A., and Wetsel,R.A. (1991). *J. Immunol.*, **146,** 362.
41. Tack,B.F., Harrison,R.A., Janatova,J., Thomas,M.L., and Prahl,J.W. (1980). *Proc. Natl Acad. Sci. USA*, **77.** 5764.

42. Sottrup-Jensen,L. (1987). In *The plasma proteins* (ed. F.W.Putnam), Vol. V, p.191. Academic Press, Florida.
43. Pangburn,M.K. and Müller-Eberhard,H.J. (1980). *J. Exp. Med.*, **152,** 1102.
44. Dodds,A.W. and Law,S.K.A. (1988). *Complement*, **5,** 89.
45. Carroll,M.C., Fathallah,D.M., Bergamaschini,L., Alicot,E.M., and Isenman,D.E. (1990). *Proc. Natl Acad. Sci. USA*, **87,** 6868.
46. Sepp,A., Dodds,A.W., Anderson,M.J., Campbell,R.D., Willis,A.C., and Law,S.K.A. (1993). *Protein Science*, **2,** 706.
47. Fielder,A.H.L., Walport,M.J., Batchelor,J.R., Rynes,R.I., Black,C.M., Dodi,I.A., and Hughes,G.R.V. (1983). *Br. Med. J. Clin. Res.*, **286**, 425.
48. Finco,O., Li,S., Cuccia,M., Rosen,F.S., and Carroll,M.C. (1992). *J. Exp. Med.*, **175**, 537.
49. Hourcade,D., Garcia,A.D., Post,T.W., Taillon-Miller,P., Holers,V.M., Wagner,L.M., Bora,N.S., and Atkinson,J.P. (1992). *Genomics*, **12,** 289.
50. Norman,D.G., Barlow,P.N., Baron,M., Day,A.J., Sim,R.B., and Campbell,R.D. (1991). *J. Mol. Biol.*, **219,** 717.
51. Dodds,A.W. and Day,A.J. (1993). In *Complement in health and disease* (ed. K.Whaley, M.Loos, and J.M.Weiler) p. 39. Immunology and Medicine Series 20. Kluwer Academic Publishers, London.
52. Klickstein,L.B., Wong,W.W., Smith,J.A., Weis,J.H, Wilson,J.G., and Fearon,D.T. (1987). *J. Exp. Med.*, **165,** 1095.
53. Klickstein,L.B., Bartow,T.J., Miletic,V., Rabson,L.D., Smith,J.A., and Fearon,D.T. (1988). *J. Exp. Med.*, **168,** 1699.
54. Moore,M.D., Cooper,N.R., Tack,B.F., and Nemerow,G.R. (1987). *Proc. Natl Acad. Sci. USA*, **84,** 9194.
55. Weis,J.J., Toothaker,E., Smith,J.A., Weis,J.H., and Fearon,D.T. (1988). *J. Exp. Med.*, **167,** 1047.
56. Wong,W.W., Cahill,J.M., Rosen,M.D., Kennedy,C.A., Bonaccio,E.T., Morris,M.J., Wilson,J.G., Klickstein,L.B., and Fearon,D.T. (1989). *J. Exp. Med.*, **169,** 847.
57. Ahearn,J.M. and Fearon,D.T. (1989). *Adv. Immunol.*, **46,** 183.
58. Martin,D.R., Yuryev,A., Kalli,K.R., Fearon,D.T., and Ahearn,J.M. (1991). *J. Exp. Med.*, **174,** 1299.
59. Caras,I.W., Davitz,M.A., Rhee,L., Weddell,G., Martin,D.W, and Nussenzweig,V. (1987). *Nature*, **325,** 545.
60. Medof,M.E., Lublin,D.M., Holers,V.M., Ayers,D.J., Getty,R.R., Leykam,J.K., Atkinson,J.P., and Tykocinski,M.L. (1987). *Proc. Natl Acad. Sci. USA*, **84,** 2007.
61. Lublin,D.M., Liszewski,M.K., Post,T.W., Arce,M.A., Le Beau,M.M., Rebentisch,M.B., Lemons,L.S., Seya,T., and Atkinson,J.P. (1988). *J. Exp. Med.*, **168,** 181.
62. Davitz,M.A., Low,M.G., and Nussenzweig,V. (1986). *J. Exp. Med.*, **163,** 1150.
63. Liszewski,M.K., Post,T.W., and Atkinson,J.P. (1991). *Ann. Rev. Immunol.*, **9,** 431.
64. Chung,L.P., Bentley,D.R., and Reid,K.B.M. (1985). *Biochem. J.*, **230,** 133.
65. Dahlback,B., Smith,C.A., and Müller-Eberhard,H.J. (1983). *Proc. Natl Acad. Sci. USA*, **80,** 3461.
66. Hillarp,A. and Dahlbäck,B. (1990). *Proc. Natl Acad. Sci. USA*, **87,** 1183.
67. Pardo-Manuel,F., Rey-Campos,J., Hillarp,A., Dahlbäck,B., and Rodriguez de Cordoba,S. (1990). *Proc. Natl Acad. Sci. USA*, **87,** 4529.
68. Ripoche,J., Day,A.J., Harris,T.J.R., and Sim,R.B. (1988). *Biochem. J.*, **249,** 593.
69. Alsenz,J., Schulz,T.F., Lambris,J.D., Sim,R.B., and Dierich,M.P. (1985). *Biochem. J.*, **232,** 841.
70. Fearon,D.T. (1978). *Proc. Natl Acad. Sci. USA*, **75,** 1971.
71. Meri,S. and Pangburn,M.K. (1990). *Proc. Natl Acad. Sci. USA*, **87,** 3982.

72. Estaller,C., Schwaeble,W., Dierich,M., and Weiss,E.H. (1991). *Eur. J. Immunol.*, **21**, 799.
73. Zipfel,P.F. and Skerka,C. (1994). *Immunol. Today*, **15**, 121.
74. DiScipio,R.D. and Hugli,T.E. (1989). *J. Biol. Chem.*, **264**, 16197.
75. Haefliger,J.A., Tschopp,J., Vial,N., and Jenne,D.E. (1989). *J. Biol. Chem.*, **264**, 18041.
76. DiScipio,R.G., Chakravarti,D.N., Müller-Eberhard,H.J., and Fey,G.H. (1988). *J. Biol. Chem.*, **263**, 549.
77. Rao,A.G., Howard,O.M.Z., Ng,S.C., Whitehead,A.S., Colten,H.R., and Sodetz,J.M. (1987). *Biochemistry*, **26**, 3556.
78. Haefliger,J.A., Tschopp,J., Naedelli,D., Wahli,W., Kocher,H.P., Tosi,M., and Stanley,K.K. (1987). *Biochemistry*, **26**, 3551.
79. Howard,O.M.Z., Rao,A.G., and Sodetz,J.M. (1987). *Biochemistry*, **26**, 3565.
80. Stanley,K.K., Kocher,H.P., Luzio,J.P., Jackson,P., and Tschopp,J. (1985). *EMBO J.*, **4**, 374.
81. Lichtenheld,M.G., Olsen,K.J., Lu,P., Lowrey,D.M., Hameed,A., Hengartner,H., and Podack,E.R. (1988). *Nature*, **325**, 448.
82. Podack,E.R. (1985). *Immunol. Today*, **6**, 21.
83. Podack,E.R. and Tschopp,J. (1982). *Proc. Natl Acad. Sci. USA*, **79**, 574.
84. Haefliger,J.A., Jenne,D., Stanley,K.K., and Tschopp,J. (1987). *Biochem. Biophys. Res. Commun.*, **149**, 750.
85. Podack,E.R. (1986). In *Immunobiology of the complement system* (ed. G.D.Ross), p. 115. Academic Press, London.
86. Jenne,D. and Stanley,K.K. (1985). *EMBO J.*, **4**, 3153.
87. Jenne,D.E. and Tschopp,J. (1989). *Proc. Natl Acad. Sci. USA*, **86**, 7123.
88. Kirszbaum,L., Sharpe,J.A., Murphy,B., d'Apice,A.J., Classon,B., Hudson,P., and Walker,I.D. (1989). *EMBO J.*, **8**, 711.
89. O'Bryan,M.K., Baker,H.W., Saunders,J.R., Kirszbaum,L., Walker,I.D., Hudson,P., Liu,D.Y., Glew,M.D., d'Apice,A.J., and Murphy,B.F. (1990). *J. Clin. Invest.*, **85**, 1477.
90. Davies,A., Simmons,D.L., Hale,G., Harrison,R.A., Tighe, H., Lachmann,P.J., and Waldmann,H. (1989). *J. Exp. Med.*, **170**, 637.
91. Lachmann,P.J. (1991). *Immunol. Today*, **12**, 312.
92. Rooney,I.A., Atkinson,J.P., Krul,E.S., Schonfeld,G., Polakoski,K., Saffitz,J.E., and Morgan,B.P. (1993). *J. Exp. Med.*, **177**, 1409.
93. Morgan,B.P. (1993). In *Complement in health and disease* (ed. K.Whaley, M.Loos, and J.M.Weiler), p. 325. Immunology and Medicine Series 20. Kluwer Academic, London.
94. Nolan,K.F., Kaluz,S., Higgins,J.M.G., Goundis,D., and Reid,K.B.M. (1992). *Biochem. J.*, **287**, 291.
95. Lawler,J. and Hynes,R.O. (1986). *J. Cell Biol.*, **103**, 1635.
96. Goundis,D. and Reid,K.B.M. (1988). *Nature*, **335**, 82.
97. Law,S.K., Fearon,D.T., and Levine,R.P. (1979). *J. Immunol.*, **122**, 759.
98. Hynes,R.O. (1992). *Cell*, **69**, 11.
99. Larson,R.S. and Springer,T.A. (1990). *Immunol. Rev.*, **144**, 181.
100. Kishimoto,T.K., O'Connor,K., Lee, A., Roberts,T.M., and Springer, T.A. (1987). *Cell*, **48**, 681.
101. Law,S.K.A., Gagnon,J., Hildreth,J.E.K., Wells,C.E., Willis,A.C., and Wong,A.J. (1987). *EMBO J.*, **6**, 915.
102. Larson,R.S., Corbi,A.L., Berman,L., and Springer,T. (1989). *J. Cell. Biol.*, **108**, 703.
103. Arnaout,M.A., Gupta,S.K., Pierce,M.W., and Tenen,D.G. (1988). *J. Cell Biol*, **106**, 2153.

104. Corbi,A.L., Kishimoto,T.K., Miller,L.J., and Springer,T.A. (1988). *J. Biol. Chem.*, **263,** 12403.
105. Hickstein,D.D., Hickey,M.J., Ozols,J., Baker,D.M., Back,A.L., and Roth,G.J. (1989). *Proc. Natl Acad. Sci. USA*, **86,** 257.
106. Corbi,A.L., Miller,L.J., O'Connor,K., Larson,R.S., and Springer,T.A. (1987). *EMBO J.*, **6,** 4023.
107. Springer,T.A. (1994). *Cell*, **76,** 301.
108. Weitzman,J.B. and Law,S.K.A. (1993). In *Complement in health and disease* (ed. K.Whaley, M.Loos, and J.M.Weiler), p. 269. Immunology and Medicine Series 20. Kluwer Academic, London.
109. Micklem,K.J. and Sim,R.B. (1985). *Biochem. J.*, **231,** 233.
110. Malhotra,V., Hogg,N., and Sim,R.B. (1986). *Eur. J. Immunol.*, **16,** 1117.
111. Gerard,N.P. and Gerard,C. (1991). *Nature*, **349,** 614.
112. Boulay,F., Mery,L., Tardif,M., Brouchon,L., and Vignais,P. (1991). *Biochemistry*, **30,** 2993.
113. Rollins,T.E., Siciliano,S., Kobayashi,S., Cianciarulo,D.N., Bonilla-Argudo,V., Collier,K., and Springer,M.S. (1991). *Proc. Natl Acad. Sci. USA*, **88,** 971.
114. Boulay,F., Tardif,M., Brouchan,L., and Vignais,P. (1990). *Biochemistry*, **29,** 11123.
115. Lu,J.H., Thiel,S., Wiedemann,H., Timpl,R., and Reid,K.B.M. (1990). *J. Immunol.*, **144,** 2287.
116. Lu,J., Wiedemann,H., Holmskov,U., Thiel,S., Timpl,R., and Reid,K.B.M. (1993). *Eur. J. Biochem.*, **215,** 793.
117. Bristow,J., Gitelman,S.E., Tee,M.K., Staels, B., and Miller,W.L. (1993). *J. Biol. Chem.*, **268,** 12919.
118. Hauptmann,G., Goetz,J., Uring-Lambert,B., and Grosshans,E. (1986). *Prog. Allergy*, **39,** 232.

4

Role of complement in health and disease

1. Biosynthesis of complement components

Most soluble complement components, with the exception of C1q, factor D, properdin, and C7 are primarily synthesized in the liver. Extrahepatic biosynthesis of most components has also been reported. In addition to contributing to the circulating pool, complement proteins produced at extrahepatic sites are thought to serve as a source for local responses to immunological challenges.

Complement proteins are modest acute-phase proteins. Plasma levels of complement components may increase by up to two- or three-fold with the onset of inflammation, probably due to their increased biosynthesis in the liver. Experiments with hepatocyte cultures show a similar increase in complement protein secretion when induced with various mediators of inflammation including tumour necrosis factor (TNF), interleukin-1 (IL-1), and interleukin-6 (IL-6) (1, 2). Local response to inflammatory mediators may vary with the cell types involved. It has been observed that skin-derived fibroblasts, when exposed to IL-1 and TNF, may increase the production of factor B by over 100-fold and C3 by about 15-fold (3).

Although the primary source of serum C1q has also not been unequivocally identified it seems likely, from cell culture and Northern blotting studies, that macrophages are the major site of C1q biosynthesis (4). In addition to secreting C1q, macrophages also appear to display the molecule on their cell surface where it may be involved in various cellular events such as binding of the Fc region of IgG, polyanions, and the lipid A portion of LPS Gram-negative bacteria (5).

The major site of biosynthesis of human serum properdin has not been established, but macrophages have been shown to synthesize properdin in *in vitro* studies and cDNA clones for both human and mouse properdin have been isolated from libraries constructed from macrophage RNA (6, 7). As judged by Northern blotting studies, the spleen may be the major organ involved in biosynthesis of properdin, with very little biosynthesis taking place in the liver (6, 8).

The major cell type responsible for factor D biosynthesis is probably the adipocyte present in fat tissue (9) although its biosynthesis has also been observed in various types of macrophages. In addition to being a complement protein, factor D probably also plays some part in fat metabolism and the murine molecule was first described as adipsin before its identity as factor D was established.

Making use of an allotypic polymorphism, the type of C7 produced by the recipient and the donor of a liver transplant could be distinguished. It was found that C7 in the patient's circulation was of the allotype of the recipient, thus suggesting that the major site of C7 biosynthesis is not the liver (10). Other terminal complement proteins, namely C6, C8, and C9, are synthesized predominantly in the liver.

Most of the membrane-bound proteins are synthesized in the cell on which they are expressed. In a recent study, CD59, a GPI-linked protein, on spermatozoa was found to be acquired from membrane vesicles in seminal plasma (11). These vesicles, called prostasomes, also carry other GPI-linked proteins including DAF but apparently not MCP, which is a transmembrane protein. These findings indicate that expression of GPI-linked proteins are not necessarily restricted to the surface of cells in which they are synthesized, but that they could be distributed to other cells and tissues via membrane vesicles.

2. Immune complex clearance

The importance of complement in immune complex clearance is clearly evident as judged by the high incidence of immune complex disorders in people deficient in complement components of the classical activation pathway. Large lattices of interconnecting molecules can be formed when a protein or particulate antigen is exposed to an antiserum. This is due to the presence, in the antiserum, of a mixture of antibody molecules, each specific for one of the many epitopes on the antigen, and the bivalent binding properties of the antibody molecules themselves which enable the formation of a lattice of antigen–antibody molecules. (It should be noted that monoclonal antibodies against a monomeric antigen do not form large immune aggregates.) The size of the complex formed is highly dependent upon the ratio of antigen to antibody and once the complex reaches a certain size, maximum precipitation occurs. When antibody is in excess precipitation still occurs, but when antigen is in excess soluble complexes are formed. Studies carried out *in vitro* show that the precipitation can be inhibited using serum by means of the functional components of the classical pathway (*Figure 4.1*). This inhibition can be abolished by the removal of one of these components, or by heating at 56°C for 30 min, or by the addition of ethylenediaminetetraacetate (EDTA) (12). Heating to 56°C causes the denaturation of certain complement components such as C1q and factor B, and EDTA chelates the divalent cations thus destabilizing the C1 complex, which requires Ca^{2+}, and inhibiting the formation of the C3 and C5 convertases, which require Mg^{2+}. When the antibody–antigen complex reaches a certain size, it activates the complement components C1, C4, C2, and C3. When sufficient C3b molecules are covalently

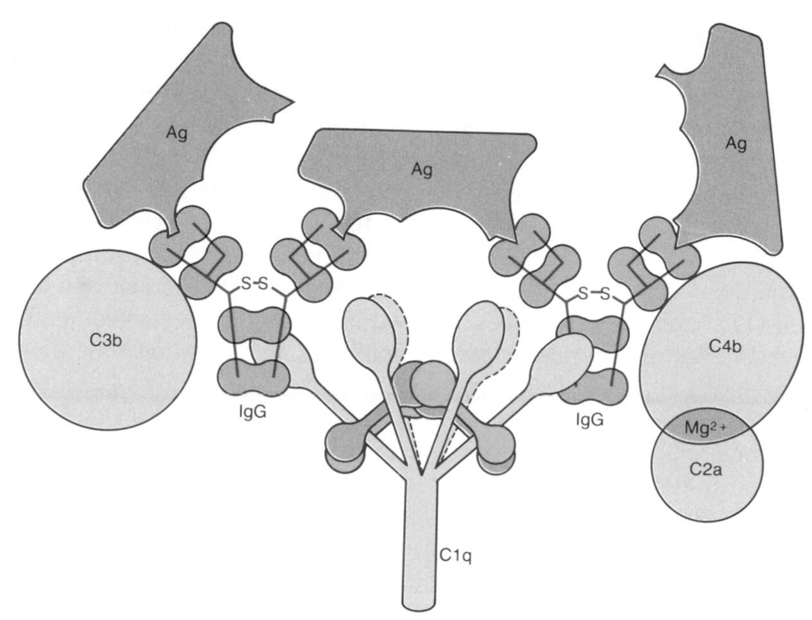

Figure 1.1. Interaction of the early classical complement components with antibody–antigen (Ag) complexes. Interaction of the C1 complex ($C1q{-}C1r_2{-}C1s_2$) with antibody IgG, by the binding of the heads of C1q to the C_H2 domain of the Fc region of the immunoglobulin, allows activation of the C1r and C1s pro-enzymes to take place. The activated C1s, in the bound C1 complex, continues activation by splitting C4 into C4a and C4b and C2 into C2a and C2b. The C4b2a complex, in the presence of Mg^{2+}, is the C3-convertase which splits C3 into C3a and C3b. A small percentage of the freshly activated C4b and C3b becomes covalently bound to the Fd regions (N-terminal halves of the heavy chains) of the antibody molecule. It is thought that the covalent binding of C3b and C4b to IgG prevents the unlimited growth of the immune complex resulting in immunoprecipitation. In addition, the C3b-coated immune complexes are able to bind to the CR1 of erythrocytes, which carry the immune complexes to the liver and spleen where they are ingested by macrophages. Complement activation is also controlled by the C1-Inh, which combines stoichiometrically with C1r and C1s, removing them from the antibody–antigen aggregate thus leaving the collagen-like regions of C1q free to interact with suitable receptors found on a wide variety of cells (see *Table 1.3*).

bound to the antigen–antibody complex, further growth of the lattice is arrested. Since C3-deficient serum does not inhibit the precipitation reaction, the role of the earlier components, in this biological function, appears to be primarily concerned with the efficient activation of C3 (13). Serum deficient in the alternative pathway components, namely properdin and factors D or B, are effective in preventing the formation of immune precipitates, suggesting that the alternative pathway does not play a major role. However, it has been observed, in *in vitro* studies, that the deposition of C3b via the alternative pathway, on pre-formed immune complexes, leads to their solubilization (14). Again, it is thought that the covalent deposition of C3b is the key to the solubilization process. Up to one C3b molecule per IgG molecule is found in the solubilized complexes. A significant proportion of the C3b molecules are bound to the Fd region of the IgG molecule.

Complement-bearing immune complexes are able to bind receptors specific for the activation fragments of complement proteins C3 and C4. In primates, CR1 on erythrocytes is the most abundant receptor for C3b and C4b in the blood. Immune complexes are transported on erythrocytes to the liver and spleen where they are cleared, presumably by the resident macrophages in these organs (15, 16). This clearance pathway was demonstrated when pre-formed labelled immune complexes were infused into the aorta of baboons and their fate followed (17). Immune complexes, infused into baboons decomplemented with cobra venom factor, are also cleared rapidly from circulation, but they were found to deposit in tissues including the heart, lung, and kidney where they have the potential to cause tissue damage (18). CR1 also serves as a cofactor for the factor-I mediated cleavage of C3b into iC3b, which has very low affinity for CR1. It should be noted that activation of complement is a continual process. Fresh C3b is continuously deposited on the immune complexes to provide the means of adhesion to CR1. Ultimately, iC3b on the immune complexes will serve as the ligand for CR3 on macrophages when the immune complexes are stripped off the erythrocytes and ingested. Animals other than primates do not have CR1 on their erythrocytes. Instead, CR1 is found on platelets, which have been shown to be the vehicles for the transport of immune complexes in these animals (19). The role of complement in immune complex clearance is summarized in *Figure 4.2*.

When considering immune complex disease in the general population then, of course, the majority of patients are not completely deficient in any of the early components of the complement system. The types of immune complex disease are quite varied, for example rheumatoid arthritis (where an inflammatory response may be brought about by presence of antibody–antigen complexes in the synovial fluid); types of glomerulonephritis (due to trapping of complexes within the glomerulus or the binding of antibody to antigens in the glomerulus); extrinsic allergic alveolitis (as in 'farmer's lung' where the antigens are inhaled); filariasis (where antigens may be released from parasites on the lymphatic vessels); and erythema nodosum (where chemotherapy of patients with high levels of antibody against the leprosy bacillus results in antigen release and immune complex formation). In these types of patients more subtle 'defects' of the complement system may play a role, for example the sera from individuals who lack the C4A isotype are found to be more susceptible to systemic lupus erythematosus (SLE) (20). This could possibly be explained by the higher covalent binding efficiency of C4A, compared to that of C4B, to immune complexes (21) thus enhancing their binding to erythrocyte CR1 and subsequent clearance (22). General reduction of complement levels may also contribute to immune complex formation. Likewise, conditions which raise levels of any serum proteins that can have an inhibitory role in the initial interaction of the classical pathway with immune complexes could predispose an individual to immune complex disease. It is also possible for pathological events to exacerbate the effects of complement activa-

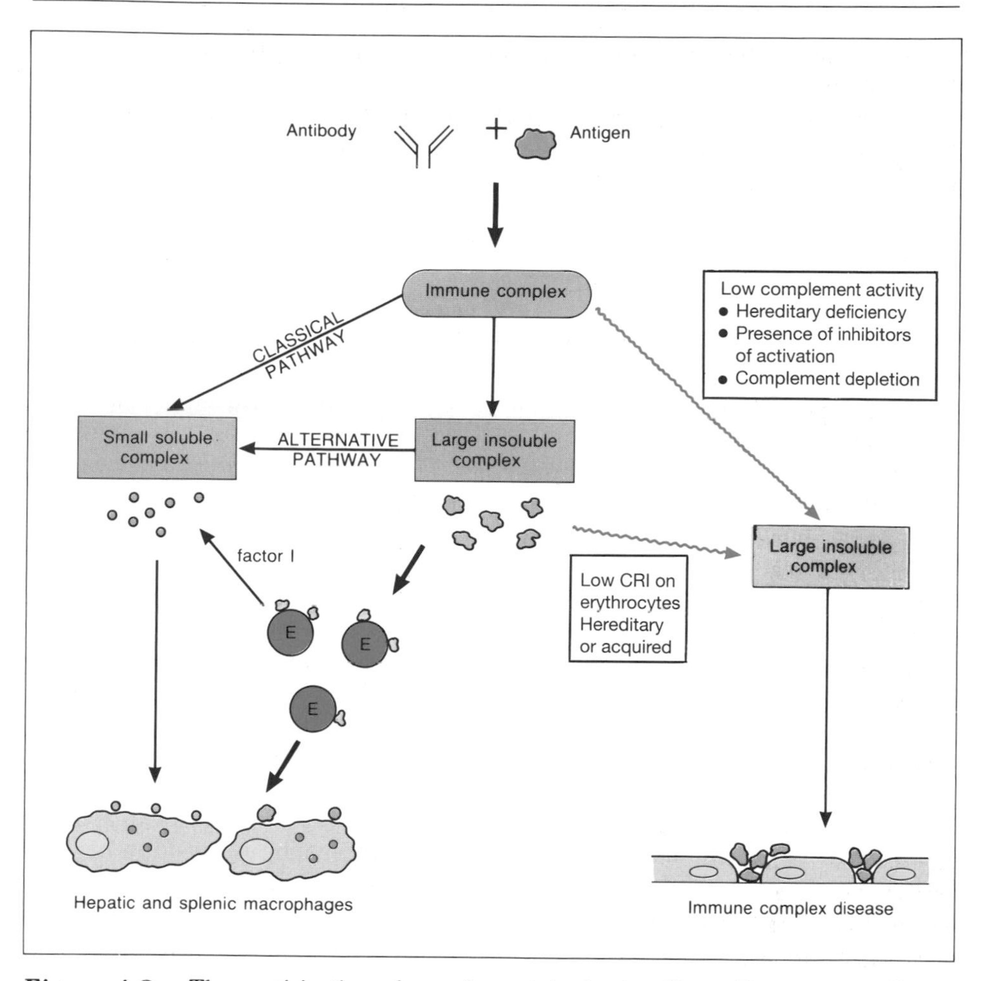

Figure 4.2. The participation of complement in the handling of immune complexes (adapted from ref. 80). The classical pathway prevents the formation of large insoluble complexes. However, in the cases when large insoluble complexes do form, the alternative pathway could be activated when such complexes reach a certain size. Covalent binding of C3b leads to the breaking up of the Ab–Ag matrix into small soluble complexes. Small complexes are cleared by hepatic and splenic macrophages. Large insoluble complexes require the binding to CR1 on erythrocytes (E) and they are transported to the liver and spleen, where they are cleared. If complement activity is subnormal for any number of reasons (e.g. due to the hereditary deficiency of a complement component, the presence of inhibitors of activation, or the depletion of complement in disease) or if CR1 on erythrocytes is low, either as a hereditary trait or acquired under disease conditions, the insoluble complexes are not efficiently transported to the liver and spleen but are deposited in other organs and tissues resulting in inflammation at these sites.

tion in immune complex disease. An example is the production of C3 nephritic factor (C3NeF) in some patients with membranoproliferative glomerulonephritis. C3NeF is an auto-antibody which binds to and stabilizes the alternative pathway C3-convertase, thereby potentiating C3 deposition in kidney glomeruli, via the alternative pathway (23).

3. Inflammation

Inflammation is the body's response to tissue damage and injury and is mediated by several interconnected plasma enzyme cascades, including complement. Inflammatory mediators are also released by resident cells in tissues, such as mast cells, as well as by cells recruited from the blood stream, such as activated monocytes and neutrophils. The involvement of complement in inflammation is mainly by the two anaphylatoxins C3a and C5a, which are the small fragments of 77 and 74 amino acids derived from the N-termini of the α chains of the two parent molecules C3 and C5, respectively. Both are spasmogenic with C5a being about 20 times as potent as C3a. C4a has also been described as anaphylatoxic, but it is only about 1% as active as C3a and is therefore probably not important in the inflammatory response *in vivo*. The spasmogenic activity of C3a and C5a requires their C-terminal Arg residue. Removal of the Arg by carboxypeptidase N (anaphylatoxin inactivator) abolishes their capacity to bind to receptors on mast cells. Thus their activity is restricted to the immediate locality of the site of injury. The activities of the anaphylatoxins are also regulated at the responding cells. Cells stimulated by an anaphylatoxin are refractory to the same anaphylatoxin, i.e. they became non-responsive to the same anaphylatoxin for a certain period. Since C3a and C4a cross-desensitize each other, but not C5a (24, 25), it may be assumed that C3a and C4a have a receptor different from that of C5a.

A series of inflammatory activities have been attributed to C3a and C5a. They include the induction of smooth muscle contraction, vasodilation, and increase in vascular permeability (*Figure 4.3*). Two of the well established assays, the contraction of guinea pig ileum and the permeation of dye in guinea pig skin, are based on these activities. The anaphylatoxins also induce mast cell degranulation (histamine release), platelet aggregation, IL-1 release from monocytes, and the release of prostaglandins and leukotrienes from various cells and tissues (26). These agents have an amplification effect on the observed vasoactive activities. It should be stressed that during an inflammatory response, many mediators with overlapping activities are present and their individual contributions are not always clear cut (*Figure 4.2*).

C5a is the principal chemotactic factor for phagocytes. Unlike the control of its spasmogenic activities, the removal of the Arg at the C-terminal of C5a only partially reduces its chemotactic activity. Migration of C5a from tissue into the bloodstream could also be assisted by vasodilation. The binding of C5a to blood phagocytes promotes their adhesion to endothelial cells lining the blood vessels, followed by their infiltration through the basement membrane and their chemotaxis

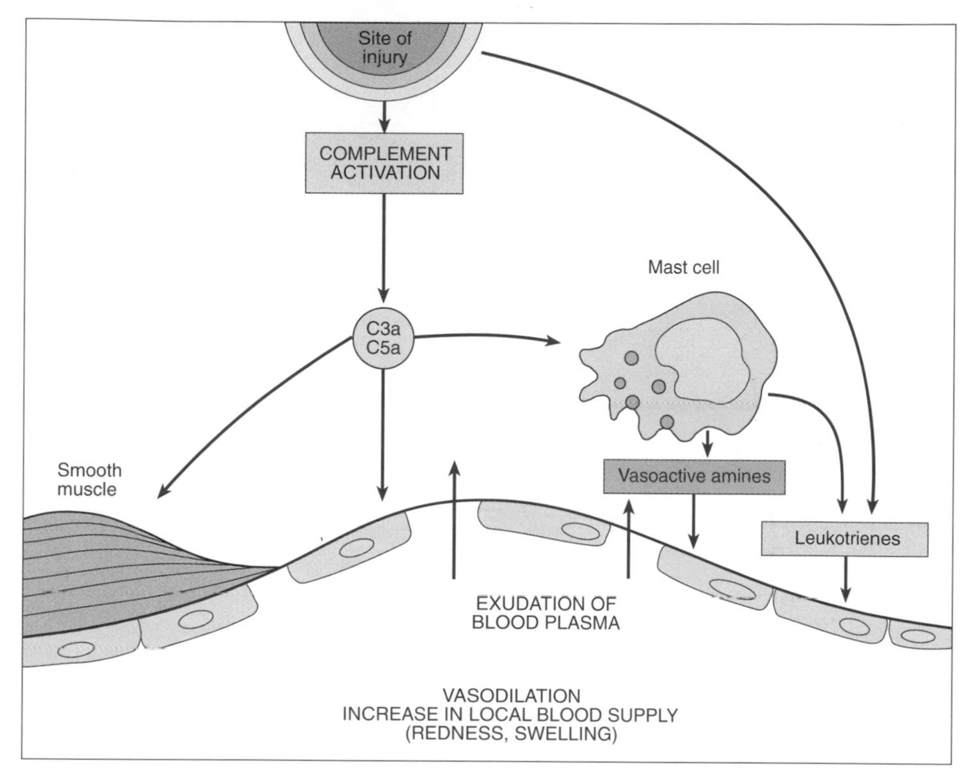

Figure 4.3. Role of complement in inflammation (I). The anaphylatoxins induce the smooth muscle of the vessel walls to contract, resulting in the local dilation of blood vessels. Stress on the endothelial lining also allows the exudation of blood plasma into the tissue. The anaphylatoxins also induce resident mast cells to release vasoactive amines (histamine) and leukotrienes which amplify the effects of the anaphylatoxins.

towards the site of injury up a concentration gradient of C5a (27). A set of cellular responses is also evident: (i) an internal pool of complement receptors, both CR1 and CR3, and possibly the p150,95 antigen, are mobilized to the cell surface from intracellular granules, and this could be the direct cause of adherence of phagocytes to the endothelium (28); (ii) the release of intracellular enzymes and leukotrienes (29, 30); and (iii) the production of toxic oxygen metabolites (31). Each of these responses could be considered as an enhancement of the cytotoxic capacity of the phagocytes. The activities of the anaphylatoxins on phagocytic cells are illustrated in *Figure 4.4*.

4. Opsonization and phagocytosis

Phagocytes, whose function is to ingest and dispose of unwanted cell debris, immune aggregates, bacteria, and other microorganisms, can only do so if they

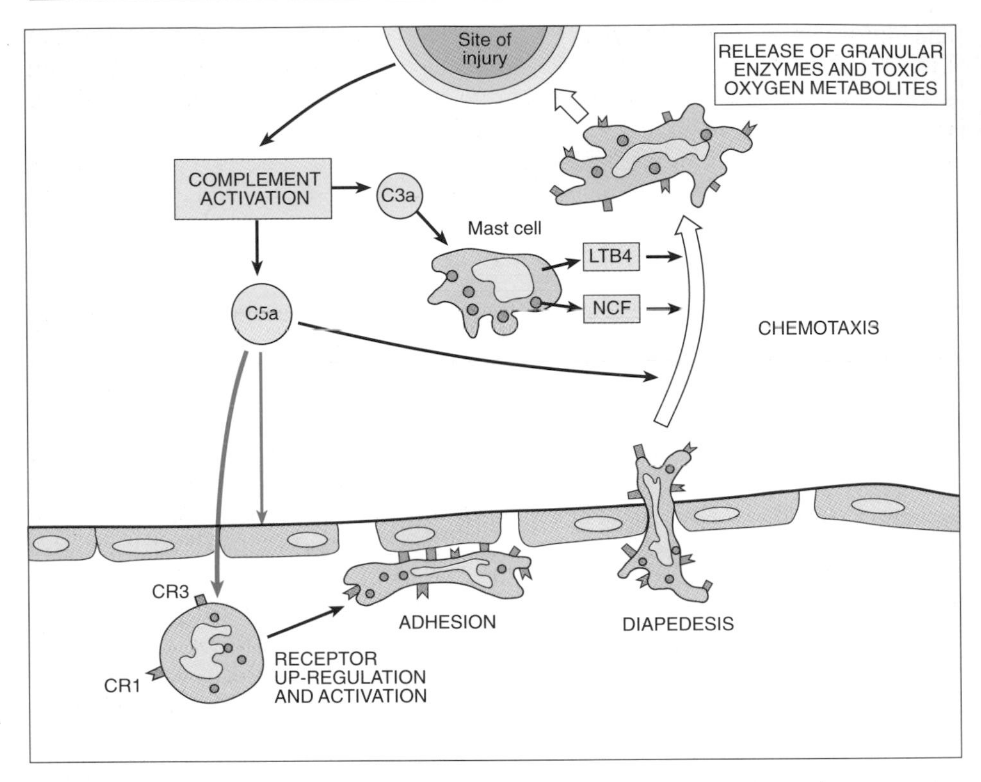

Figure 4.4. Role of complement in inflammation (II). C5a up-regulates the expression of CR1 and CR3 on phagocytes and promotes their adhesion to and subsequent transmigration across the endothelium (diapedesis). C3a and C5a also trigger resident mast cells to release various factors, which, in addition to C5a, promote chemotaxis of phagocytes towards the site of injury. They also trigger the phagocytes to release granular enzymes and produce toxic oxygen metabolites. Mast cell factors shown in the figure are leukotrine B4 (LTB4) and neutrophil chemotactic factor (NCF).

can recognize and distinguish them from host cells. The host defence therefore labels these targets with antibody and complement fragments, and the phagocytes recognize these labels by the receptors on their surfaces specific for these labels. The coating of targets with antibody and complement fragments is frequently referred to as 'opsonization', which means 'preparation for food'.

Phagocytes include the polymorphonuclear leukocytes and monocytes in the blood and cells of the monocyte/macrophage lineage in various tissues and organs. The major phagocytic receptors are the Fc receptors (FcR), which recognize the Fc portion of the IgG antibody, and the two complement receptors CR1 (which recognizes C3b and C4b) and CR3 (which recognizes iC3b).

Freshly isolated blood monocytes express all three receptors but can only ingest IgG-coated targets. The interactions via CR1 and CR3 with complement fragments serve to promote adhesion when the IgG on the target surface is low. In the presence of an appropriate second signal, cultured monocytes can bind and ingest complement-coated targets in the absence of the IgG–FcR interaction (32, 33). The second signal can be generated by the culture of monocytes on surfaces coated with fibronectin or serum amyloid P, or the treatment of the monocytes with phorbol esters which activate protein kinase C (34). These second signals may have a common effect on promoting the assembly of microtubules. Drugs promoting microtubule assembly also promote complement receptor-mediated phagocytosis and those preventing microtubule assembly have an inhibitory effect (35). In addition, these drugs do not appear to affect FcR mediated phagocytosis.

An additional role is assumed by CR3 in the ingestion phase of both FcR and CR-mediated phagocytosis. Several anti-CR3 monoclonal antibodies have been found to inhibit the ingestion of IgG-opsonized targets (36). Further work has shown that CR3 on monocytes falls into one of two subsets. Whereas the mobile subset appears to function as a complement receptor, the immobile subset, presumably by interacting with cytoskeletal elements, plays a role in the ingestion process (37). The ingestion process involves the mobilization of actin filaments to engulf the opsonized targets, and is inhibited by drugs, such as cytochalasin B, which disrupt the actin filament network (35, 38). The opsonized targets are taken up as internalized vesicles appropriately called phagosomes, which fuse with lysosomes to allow the final digestion of the target (*Figure 4.5*)

The C1q receptor which is found on a wide variety of cells such as monocytes, neutrophils, eosinophils, and endothelial cells, may play a role in the enhancement of phagocytosis by its interaction with C1q or certain collectins including MBP, conglutinin, and the lung surfactant protein A (SP-A) (39, 40). Also, triggering of the C1q receptors on neutrophils, eosinophils, or endothelial cells enhances the generation of toxic oxygen species which can play a role in the destruction of pathogens (41).

The binding of pathogens by the lectin domains of the collectins offers an antibody-independent route of recognition and clearance. The binding of MBP to *E. coli, Salmonella montevideo, S. typhimurium*, and HIV, may lead to the enhanced phagocytosis of these organisms by the C1q/collectin receptor. However, it should be borne in mind that MBP can be involved in activation of the classical pathway of complement, therefore involvement of activated C4 and C3 and use of receptors for these fragments in the phagocytosis must also be considered.

5. Lytic function

Generally the lytic function of complement is equated to the membrane attack complex (MAC) lesions seen in a model system such as the lysis of IgM-antibody coated red blood cells with a heterologous complement. This type of study, along with studies on the lysis of re-formed red blood cell 'ghosts' and artificial liposome structures, has clearly shown that a spectrum of C5b-8$(C9)_n$ complexes can be formed, which vary in the number of C9 molecules present, n lying

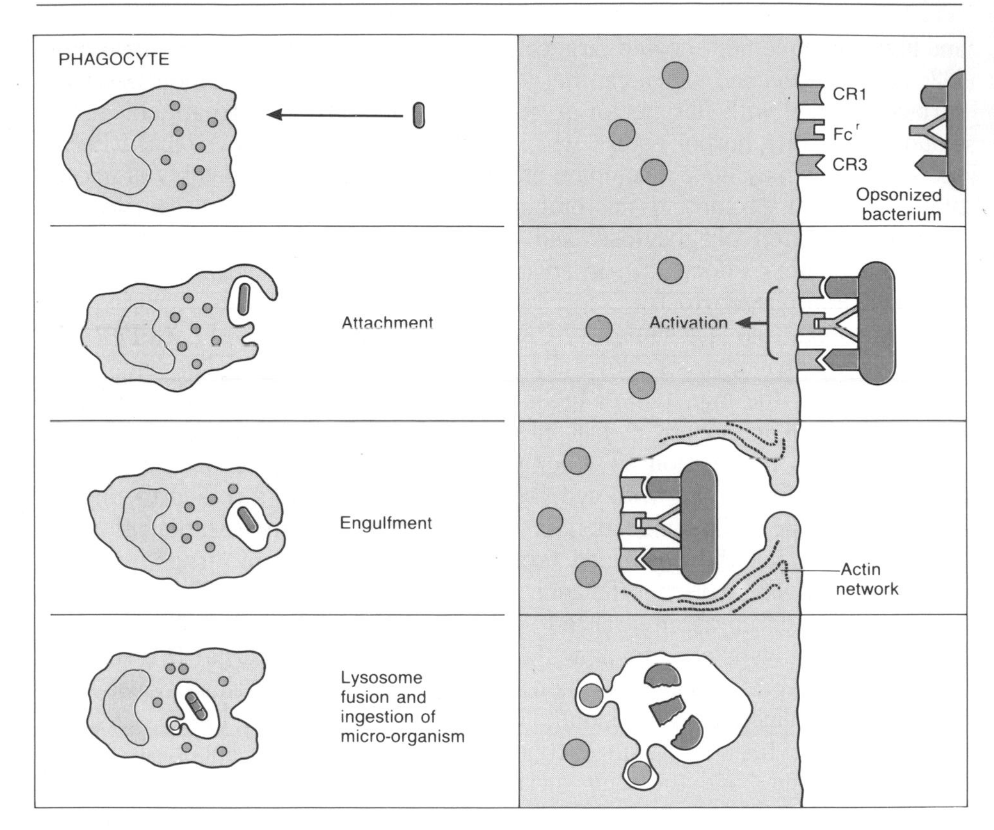

Figure 4.5. Opsonization and phagocytosis. Opsonized particles (coated with IgG, C4b, C3b, and iC3b) attach to phagocytes via CR1 (for C3b and C4b), CR3 (for iC3b), and Fc receptors (for Fc region of IgG). Binding activates the actin network to engulf the particle. The internalized vesicle is fused with lysosomes and the ingested material is digested by lysosomal enzymes

between one and 18. A MAC pore diameter of about 10 nm can be seen when 15–17 C9 molecules are present (see *Figure 2.7*) while an apparent pore size of ~3 nm has been estimated for a C5b-8$(C9)_2$ complex, and it is considered that the smaller pores will fulfil a lytic function (42). However, some of the views concerning the mode of action may have to be modified with respect to the finding that nucleated cells appear to be capable of utilizing several defence mechanisms to escape MAC attack (43). It is known that in these cells there is a rise in the concentration of intracellular free calcium ions before any cell lysis becomes detectable, and that this can activate certain cellular functions which can cause either shedding or internalization of the MAC channels and perhaps the induction of lipid repair mechanisms, thus conferring protection. Unlike a red blood cell, which probably relies only on the binding of C9 by the homologous restriction factors to inhibit attack by its own MAC, the nucleated cell is relatively resistant to complement. However, in the case of extensive complement activation (~10^5 MACs per cell) even a nucleated target cell is unlikely to survive since early pore formation by the MAC would be accompanied by the breakdown of membrane potential, with a loss of potassium and influx of sodium. The subsequent compensatory ion-pumping mechanisms along with the cell activation induced by the rise in intracellular calcium may drain the cell of energy resources and this, along with the general marked physical alteration to the cell surface, is likely to promote cell death.

In the case of the killing of Gram-negative bacteria, although there is an initial requirement for antibody to promote extensive complement activation, lysozyme also plays an important accessory role by attacking the peptidoglycan layer via the pores created by the MAC in the outer membranes. However, as in the case of nucleated cells, microorganisms have evolved a variety of mechanisms by which they can prevent opsonization and lysis by complement, and this is emphasized by the finding that pathogenic bacteria isolated from patients often exhibit increased resistance to complement. Indeed, all Gram-positive bacteria are resistant, probably as a consequence of their thick peptidoglycan layer preventing access of C5b-9 to the inner membrane (44), and nearly all fungi resist complement attack by virtue of their rigid, relatively impermeable cell wall. Some strains of Gram-negative bacteria appear to be resistant to MAC attack by limiting complement activation to a subset of lipopolysaccharide molecules bearing longer than normal *O*-polysaccharide side chains, thus sterically hindering the C5b-9 complexes from reaching the complement-sensitive sites on the outer membrane (*Figure 4.6*).

Activation of complement to the C5b-9 stage is generally beneficial to the host in fighting infection but in certain disease states, especially those of an autoimmune nature, there may be damage to host cells and tissues. For example, kidney damage in systemic lupus erythematosus (SLE) and glomerular nephritis has been partly attributed to the MAC, as has injury to motor end plates in myasthenia gravis and to the muscular microvasculature in dermatomyositis. It is possible that apart from membrane damage, sublytic doses of the MAC may

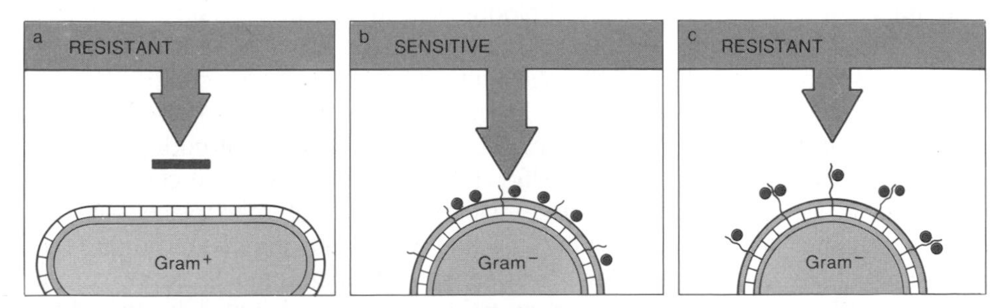

Figure 4.6. Sensitivity of bacteria to complement MAC. (**a**) Most Gram-positive ($Gram^+$) bacteria lack an outer lipid membrane and resist attack. (**b**) Some Gram-negative ($Gram^-$) bacteria are susceptible to the lytic components (orange discs) but some strains decoy the MAC by producing long antigenic filaments which cause deposition of MAC away from the outer membrane (**c**).

cause the release of toxic oxygen metabolites and arachidonic acid derivatives which may be involved in the pathogenesis of these conditions. These examples serve to emphasize the importance of mechanisms by which host cells may avoid damage by their own complement system.

6. Interaction of complement with microorganisms

The complement system is remarkable in that it can attach its activated components to, and attack, a wide variety of surfaces via hydroxyl or amino groups (covalently, through activated C4 and C3) or via membrane phospholipids through the MAC. This is amply demonstrated by considering the possible role of complement in the destruction and/or clearance of a wide variety of organisms such as Gram-negative and Gram-positive bacteria, parasites, and viruses. Specificity and recognition of these interactions is often, but not always, a function of antibody binding which usually leads to efficient complement activation.

6.1 Bacteria (45)

Complement was first described on the basis of its heat-sensitive bactericidal effect (*Figures 4.6* and *4.7*). Indeed, most Gram-negative bacteria can activate complement by both the classical and alternative pathways in the absence of antibody but efficient bacteriolysis of certain forms (the S forms) requires the bacterium to be coated with antibody. In the absence of antibody it is probably the lipopolysaccharide protein of the outer bacterial membrane which interacts directly with C1 to induce classical pathway activation and also provides a 'protected site' for the deposition of C3b, allowing formation of $\mathrm{C}\overline{\mathrm{3bBb}}$ and its protection from down regulation by factors I and H, thus allowing efficient alternative pathway activation. The membranes of complement-sensitive Gram-negative bacteria display the same type of MAC lesions as those seen in the membranes of complement-lysed red blood cells. Intact Gram-positive bacteria, on the other hand, do not activate the classical pathway in the absence of antibody, which is probably due to the quite different cell wall composition of the two classes of bacteria. However, direct activation of the alternative pathway by Gram-positive bacteria does take place, as does activation of both pathways in the presence of the binding of specific antibodies. In all cases of complement activation, lysis of the Gram-positive bacteria does not take place but the bacteria become heavily coated with C3b and iC3b, allowing opsonization (see Section 4) of the bacteria by phagocytic cells. This is an important mechanism against both Gram-positive and Gram-negative bacteria and is well illustrated by the sensitivity of C3-deficient individuals to bacterial infection.

Thus it is now recognized that the composition of the bacterial envelope is important in determining sensitivity to the lytic action of complement, with Gram-negative bacteria usually being susceptible while Gram-positive bacteria

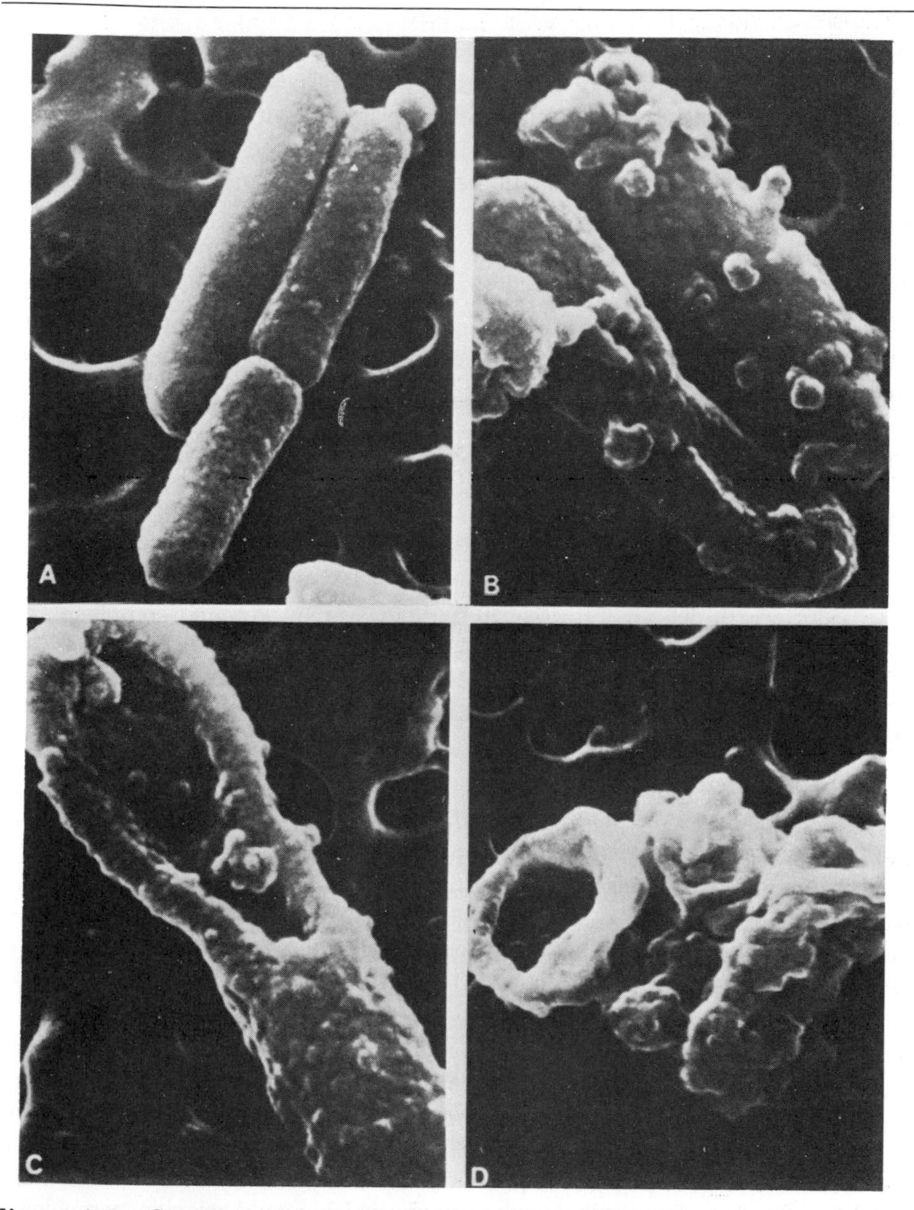

Figure 4.7. Scanning electron micrographs of *Escherichia coli* before and after killing by complement via the alternative pathway (from ref. 81 with permission). Magnification = 30 000 (**A**) Intact bacteria. (**B**) Bacteria killed by a mixture of purified alternative pathway complement components and the terminal components in the absence of lysozyme and (**C**) in the presence of lysozyme at 10 μg ml^{-1}. (**D**) Bacteria killed and lysed with C4-depleted serum. Note the increase in size of the killed bacteria and the perturbation of the protrusions on the cell surface, and the random polymorphic appearance of the killed and lysed bacteria.

are not. The composition of the bacterial membrane determines which complement pathway will be efficiently activated. It should also be noted that the surface composition of bacteria can be changed by plasmid-coded proteins which can induce resistance to complement lysis (46). In all cases the activation of complement leads to the opsonization of the bacteria.

6.2 Parasites (47)

In view of the numerous different types of parasite it is difficult to form a general overview of the possible role of complement against infection by these organisms. One feature which emerges is that many parasites appear to activate the alternative pathway of complement, and this of course would be amplified by the presence of specific antibodies. Certain flagellates such as *Leishmania* and amoebae such as *Entamoeba histolytica* show sensitivity to complement, although in the case of *Schistosomes* complement appears to offer very little defence to infection. In certain cases complement may even provide beneficial effects to the parasites, for example by allowing entry into host cells of C3b- and/or iC3b-coated parasites (*Barbesia* and *Leishmania*) via CR1 and/or CR3 on host cells. Also, side effects due to activation of complement by immune complexes can lead to host problems, such as nephritis.

6.3 Viruses (48)

Complement appears to play an important role in neutralizing viruses once the system has been activated by specific anti-viral antibodies. However, both pathways can also be triggered directly by viruses and virally infected cells without the aid of antibody. Direct activators of the classical pathway are the retroviruses Sindbis and Newcastle disease viruses, and activators of the alternative pathway are Epstein–Barr virus (EBV) and Sindbis virus. Antibody-independent activation of the alternative pathway is shown by cells infected with measles and EBV viruses. Although there is no definitive evidence that the action of complement plays a major role in recovery from viral infection it certainly appears to play an accessory role in the mechanisms of anti-viral immunity. The coating of virus particles with C4b and C3b would be expected to prevent the virus from attaching to virus cell surface receptors and to prepare the virus for phagocytosis. Perhaps, on considering its possible role in the absence of antibody, complement could be viewed as being the humoral equivalent of the natural killer cell system, which would provide some initial protection prior to the humoral and cellular immune response to a viral infection.

It has been well established that EBV uses CR2 as the receptor to gain access into B lymphocytes (49). Deliberate infection of B lymphocytes with EBV has become a standard laboratory practice to immortalize the B cells from individuals. These cells are particularly useful as a source of genetic material, for example from patients with hereditary deficiencies, for diagnosis and research purposes. Recently, it has been found that the MCP is the receptor for at least two different strains of measles virus (50, 51). It is not known if HIV-1 has molecules directly recognized by complement receptors but it can activate the classical pathway of complement in both an antibody-dependent and an antibody-independent fashion. C1q can bind directly to gp41 on the virus surface and initiate the activation of subsequent components (52). However, HIV-1 is resistant to the lytic action of human complement although it is sensitive to complement from other species. It is thought that the resistance is due to the presence on the viral surface of protective molecules, such as CD59, which is incorporated into the viral membrane as the virus matures and buds off from the infected host cell. Thus, the binding of complement fragments to the virus only serves to provide additional means for the virus to bind to host cells via the complement receptors, and complement-dependent enhancement of HIV-1 infection has been documented. For example, the enhancement of HIV-1 infection of the Raji B-cell line expressing CR2, and the U937 monocytic cell line expressing CR3, was found to be mediated via these two complement receptors respectively (53, 54). These findings have profound effects on the design of human vaccination strategies against HIV-1 since triggering of an antibody response may actually promote the susceptibility to infection (52).

7. The role of complement in the immune response

Strong indicators of complement involvement in the immune response are the findings that impairment of the immune response may be associated with deficiencies of the classical pathway components (i.e. C1, C4, and C2) and C3 both in man and in other animals. The primary response of C2- or C4-deficient guinea pigs to certain antigens is clearly depressed and repeated immunization fails to increase the response or switch the antibody isotypes from IgM to IgG (55). Injection of normal guinea pig serum, or purified human C4 protein, to C4-deficient guinea pigs at the time of primary immunization could, at least partially, restore the primary and secondary responses (56). Animals treated with cobra venom factor (CVF) are depleted of complement by continued activation of the alternative pathway. Cobra venom factor, which is cobra C3b, forms a C3-convertase which is not susceptible to control by mammalian factors H and I. These CVF-treated animals showed a marked depression of antibody responses to T-dependent antigens (57). In addition, various *in vivo* studies have also pointed to the importance of C3 in the antibody response. These studies indicated that: (i) $F(ab')_2$ anti-C3 could inhibit primary and secondary T-dependent antibody production (58, 59); (ii) C3d-K (a kallikrein cleavage fragment of iC3b) acts as an inhibitor of mitogen-induced B- and T-cell proliferation (59); and (iii) aggregated C3b or C3d can regulate the growth of activated B cells by promoting the entry of the B cells into S phase, thus enhancing division (60).

The C3 receptor on B cells is CR2, which binds iC3b and C3dg. Administration of anti-CR2 antibody to mice results in these animals showing an impaired immune response (61). Similar effects can be obtained by the introduction of recombinant soluble CR2 into mice (62). All these observations point to the importance of a C3dg–CR2 interaction in the activation of B cells. CR2 is one of the components of a multimolecular complex on the B-cell surface, two other components being the CD19 and the TAPA-1 (target for antiproliferative antibody) antigens (63). Cross-linking of surface IgM (the antigen receptor B cells) with specific antibodies causes an increase in intracellular calcium and induces B-cell proliferation. These effects can be enhanced by the addition of antibodies to the components of the CR2/CD19/TAPA-1 complex (64). CR2 and TAPA-1 have relatively small cytoplasmic domains but CD19 contains sequence motifs known to bind phosphatidyl inositol 3-kinases. It is likely that the signal transduction pathway for B-cell activation involves the co-ligation of surface IgM and the CR2/CD19/TAPA-1 complex via an intracellular phosphorylation event (63).

Other complement components and their activated fragments, including C1q, the anaphylatoxins C3a and C5a, and their des-Arg forms, have also been reported to have immunoregulatory activities. However, it appears that these activities are mostly in the stimulation of release, from various leukocytes, of other immunoregulators such as interleukins, their inhibitors, and various arachidonic acid metabolites (65, 66).

8. Complement deficiencies

Deficiencies in a number of complement proteins are well documented and patients suffer from various degrees of illness. The deficiencies can be roughly categorized into six groups: (i) the classical pathway components, (ii) the alternative pathway components; (iii) C3; (iv) the components of the MAC; (v) the regulatory proteins; and (vi) the receptors. A list of these deficiencies together with their associated major clinical symptoms can be found in *Table 4.1*.

General association can be made between the complement deficiencies and the clinical conditions of patients in the first four groups. Conclusions can therefore be drawn with regard to the function and importance of different complement components or pathways *in vivo*. The activation of C3 via the classical pathway is required in the clearance of immune complexes since deficiencies in any of the activation components (i.e. C1, C4, and C2) and C3 result in the common manifestation of immune complex disorders. It should be emphasized that in the case of C4, immune complex disorder is exclusively correlated with the deficiency of the C4A isotype, even at the level of heterozygous deficiency. Mannan binding protein, which also activates the complement cascade via C4 and C2, shows a very wide range of plasma levels (from zero to 5 $\mu g\ ml^{-1}$ with an average value of about 1 $\mu g\ ml^{-1}$ for Caucasians). Some of the variation is explained by the finding that human MBP exists in at least four allelic forms, the wild-type A form and the variant B, C, and D forms. Each of the variants is caused by a single point mutation which results in an amino acid substitution within the collagen-like region of the molecule. These substitutions are considered to interfere with the correct folding of the triple-helical region of MBP. Thus, individuals homozygous for the B, C, and D alleles have no MBP in their sera, as judged by both functional and immunochemical tests. Normal MBP can be found in the sera of heterozygous individuals who have one A allele and one of the variant alleles, but the levels are low due to the negative contribution from the defective chains produced by the B, C, or D alleles. The frequency of the alleles varies with ethnic groups; Caucasian frequencies are 0.81 for A, 0.13 for B, 0.02 for C, and 0.05 for D while in Africans values of 0.69 (A), 0.03 (B), 0.24 (C), and 0.05 (D) are found (67). However, all the low levels of MBP which are observed do not appear to be due to mutations leading to structural defects, and other factors, such as the presence of genomic elements controlling expression of the normal protein, must be considered, especially as a wide variation in MBP levels (0.13 $\mu g\ ml^{-1}$ to 5 $\mu g\ ml^{-1}$) is seen in the sera of Caucasians who are homozygous for the A allele. It is clear that young children with low MBP levels show an increased risk of suffering from recurrent infections and opsonin deficiency. This indicates that the lectin mediated pathway of complement activation may be of considerable importance for opsonization in those with immature or deficient immune systems (68).

Deficiency in factor B has not been described and it has been suggested that the deficiency is probably fatal. Deficiencies in properdin and factor D illustrate the importance of the alternative pathway in combating *Meningococcal* and *Neisserial* infections. Genetic deficiency of properdin is an X-linked recessive trait and carries a high risk of fatal fulminant *Meningococcal* infections. This illustrates the important role of properdin in ensuring that continued and efficient activation of the alternative pathway takes place (via stabilization of the enzyme complexes $\overline{C3bBb}$ and $\overline{C3b_2Bb}$ by properdin). This allows the pathogen, targeted by the alternative pathway, to be efficiently lysed by large numbers of the MAC and also to be extensively coated with C3b to allow rapid clearance. Homozygous deficiency of factor D/adipsin is very rare but in the cases which have been reported the patients usually show susceptibility to recurrent *Neisserial* infections. C3 deficient individuals have recurrent infections, the severity of which usually overshadows their impairment in immune complex clearance.

Deficiencies in the terminal complex components are correlated with susceptibility to recurrent *Neisserial* infection possibly because of the ability of these microorganisms to survive as intracellular parasites in phagocytes. Thus, the lytic activity of complement is required for their clearance. Individuals deficient in C9, however, are mostly healthy, suggesting that the four components, C5–C8, are sufficient to cause significant membrane damage and cell death.

Deficiencies in the control proteins usually result in the consumption of complement components which are normally protected from non-specific activation. Deficiency in the C1-inhibitor (C1-Inh) allows $C\overline{1s}$ to deplete C4 and C2 levels in serum and it is believed that hereditary angio-oedema, generally associated with C1-Inh deficiency, could be caused by the increase of a C2 breakdown product (69). Deficiency in factor I allows the alternative pathway to accelerate into the positive feedback loop in the fluid phase, thus depressing the level of both factor B and C3. Consequently, these patients generally suffer from bacterial infection due to the low opsonic activity brought about via the alternative

Table 4.1 Complement deficiencies

Protein	Remarks	Relative frequencies[a]	Major clinical disorder	Minor clinical disorder
Classical complement components				
C1q		Medium	Immune complex diseases	Recurrent infection
C1r		Low	SLE, glomerulonephritis	Recurrent infection
C1s		Low	SLE	
C4		Medium	Immune complex diseases	Recurrent infection
C2		High	SLE	Recurrent infection
MBP		Very high		Infections in childhood
Alternative pathway components				
B		Very rare	(May be fatal)	
D		Low	Recurrent upper respiratory infection	
P		Low	Severe meningitis	
C3				
C3		Medium	Recurrent infection	Immune complex disease
Membrane attack complex				
C5		Medium	Recurrent neisserial infection	SLE
C6		Medium	Recurrent neisserial infection	SLE

C7		Medium	Recurrent neisserial infection	SLE
C8		Medium	Recurrent neisserial infection	SLE
C9	Good health			
Control proteins				
C1-Inh	Low C4 and C2 levels	Very high	Angioedema	SLE
Factor I	Low C3 and factor B levels, no alternative pathway activity	Low	Recurrent infection	
Factor H	Partial (10%)	Low	Haemolytic uraemic syndrome	
Membrane proteins				
CR1[b]			Immune complex disorder	
CR3	Defective in β-subunit, patients also deficient in LFA-1 and 150,95	Medium	Recurrent pyogenic infection	
DAF[c]			Paroxysmal nocturnal haemoglobinuria	
CD59[c]			Paroxysmal nocturnal haemoglobinuria	

[a] The levels are arbitrarily denoted as low (<10), medium (10–15), high (50–250), and very high (>250) according to the number of cases reported. The numbers are partly based on a report in ref. 82. These data are intended to give relative frequencies among the complement deficiencies.
[b] May not be a true deficiency. Level of erythrocyte CR1 may be regulated by closely linked genetic element. Low level of CR1 may also be required in patients with SLE, rheumatoid arthritis, autoimmune haemolytic anaemia, AIDS, and paroxysmal nocturnal haemoglobinuria (PNH).
[c] Also defective in patients with deficiencies in the biosynthesis of the glycosyl phosphatidylinositol (GPI) linker.

pathway. Deficiencies in factor H and decay accelerating factor are less damaging clinically since their functional activities are also mediated by other molecules, for example CR1. Paroxysmal noctural haemoglobinuria (PNH) has long been known to correlate with the elevated sensitivity of the patients' erythrocytes to complement. Most of these patients were found to be defective in a protein involved with the synthesis of the phosphatidylinositol linker (70) and they are deficient in DAF, CD59, and other GPI-anchored membrane proteins. In one case, PNH symptoms were observed in a patient with a defect in the CD59 gene (71). It is therefore suggestive that PNH is primarily due to the absence of the lysis inhibitory molecule CD59. Deficiency in CR3 is invariably due to a defect in the β subunit (72). These patients are therefore also deficient in the two other membrane molecules LFA-1 and p150,95. The leukocytes of these patients have defective adhesion properties including their traffic between blood and tissues and the ingestion of opsonized pathogens. These patients suffer from recurrent pyogenic infections.

9. Clinical applications

Activation of complement is a key response in our fight against infection and other immunological challenges. On the other hand, activation of complement in many autoimmune and inflammatory diseases clearly brings about reactions leading to tissue damage either directly by the MAC of complement or indirectly by leukocytes responding to the signals generated by complement activation. It is therefore of medical interest to minimize complement activation in clinical procedures including blood transfusion, haemodialysis, and organ transplantation. For example, it has been shown that different natural and synthetic polymers used in the manufacture of various biomedical material, such as membrane for haemodialysis, have different capacities from active complement (73).

Anti-complement antibodies have been shown to be effective in modulating complement activities. The antibody response to T-cell dependent antigens can be suppressed, to varying degrees and depending on the immunizing dose of the antigens, by the introduction of an anti-CR2 antibody or a soluble form of CR2 (i.e. recombinant CR2 without the transmembrane and cytoplasmic regions) (61, 62). A soluble CR1 molecule produced by recombinant DNA technology has been shown to be effective in inhibiting complement activation and consequent inflammatory activities in a rat model of reperfusion injury of transient myocardial ischaemia (74). Antibodies to CR3 have been shown to inhibit the infiltration of monocytes and neutrophils to the sites of various inflammatory challenges (75, 76). However, the inhibition is likely to be directed to the adhesion properties of CR3 rather than its role as a complement receptor.

Recent work on xenotransplantation has shown that the hyperacute phase of rejection is mediated by antibody and complement. Depletion of antibody and complement in the recipient (baboon) has increased the survival time of the transplanted organ (pig heart) from 90 min to over 15 days (77). Complement activation can also be controlled by the introduction of soluble CR1 as demonstrated by the prolonged survival of guinea pig xenograft in rats (78). *In vitro* studies have shown that transfection of human proteins DAF and MCP to swine endothelial cells offers protection from human complement activities (79). These lines of research open up the possibility of producing transgenic animals with the appropriate complement regulatory proteins as a source of organs suitable for xenotransplantation.

10. Further reading

10.1 Biosynthesis of complement components

Colten,H.R. and Strunk,P.C. (1993). In *Complement in health and disease* (2nd edn) (ed. K.Whaley, M.Loos, and J.M.Weiler), p. 127. Immunology and Medicine Series 20. Kluwer Academic, London.

10.2 Immune complex clearance

Ng,Y.C. and Schifferli,J.A. (1993). In *Complement in health and disease* (2nd edn) (ed. K.Whaley, M.Loos, and J.M.Weiler), p. 199. Immunology and Medicine Series 20. Kluwer Academic, London.

Whaley,K. (1987). In *Complement in health and disease* (ed. K. Whaley), p. 163. MTP, Lancaster.

10.3 Inflammation

Köhl,J. and Bitter-Suermann,D. (1993). In *Complement in health and disease* (2nd edn) (ed. K.Whaley, M.Loos, and J.M.Weiler), p. 299. Immunology and Medicine Series 20. Kluwer Academic, London. p. 299.

Gallin,J.I. (1993). In *Fundamental Immunology* (3rd edn) (ed. W.E.Paul), p. 1015. Raven, New York.

10.4 Opsonization and phagocytosis

Weitzman,J.B. and Law,S.K.A. (1993). In *Complement in health and disease* (2nd edn) (ed. K.Whaley, M.Loos, and J.M.Weiler), p. 269. Immunology and Medicine Series 20. Kluwer Academic, London.

Greenberg,S. and Silverstein,S.C. (1993). In *Fundamental immunology* (3rd edn) (ed. W.E.Paul), p. 941. Raven, New York.

10.5 Lytic function

Morgan,B.P. (1993). In *Complement in health and disease* (2nd edn) (ed. K.Whaley, M.Loos, and J.M.Weiler), p. 325. Immunology and Medicine Series 20. Kluwer Academic, London.

10.6 Complement and microorganisms

Moffitt,M.C. and Frank,M.M. (1994). In *Seminars in immunopathology* (ed. P.J.Lachmann), Vol. 15, p. 327. Springer, Berlin.

Fishelson,Z. (1994). In *Seminars in immunopathology* (ed. P.J.Lachmann), Vol. 15, p. 345. Springer, Berlin.

10.7 *Complement and the immune response*

Fearon,D.T. (1993). *Curr. Opinion Immunol.,* **5,** 341.
Kinoshita,T. (1993). *Complement Today,* **1,** 46.

10.8 *Complement deficiencies*

Rosen,F.S. (1993). In *Complement in health and disease* (2nd edn) (ed. K.Whaley, M.Loos, and J.M.Weiler), p. 159. Immunology and Medicine Series 20. Kluwer Academic, London.
Densen,P. (1993). In *Complement in health and disease* (2nd edn) (ed. K.Whaley, M.Loos, and J.M.Weiler), p. 173, Immunology and Medicine Series 20. Kluwer Academic, London.

10.9 *Clinical applications*

Kalli,K.R., Hsu,P. and Fearon,D.T. (1994). In *Seminars in immunopathology* (ed. P.J.Lachmann), Vol. 15, p. 417. Springer, Berlin.

11. References

1. Perlmutter,D.H., Goldberger,G., Dinarello,C.A., Mizel,S.B., and Colten,H.R. (1986). *Science,* **232,** 850.
2. Perlmutter,D.H., Dinarello,C.A. Punsal,P.I., and Colten,H.R. (1986). *J. Clin. Invest.*, **78,** 1349.
3. Katz,Y. and Strunk,R.C. (1989). *J. Immunol.,* **142,** 3862.
4. Müller,W., Hanauska-Abel,H., and Loos,M. (1978). *J. Immunol.*, **121,** 1578.
5. Loos,M., Martin,H., and Petry,F. (1984). *Behring Inst. Mitt.*, **84,** 32.
6. Goundis,D. and Reid,K.B.M. (1988). *Nature,* **335,** 82.
7. Nolan,K.F., Schwaeble,W., Kaluz,S., Dierich,M.P., and Reid,K.B.M. (1991). *Eur. J. Immunol.*, **21,** 771.
8. Farries,T.C. and Atkinson,J.P. (1989). *J. Immunol.*, **142,** 842.
9. Cook,K.S., Min,H.Y., Johnson,D., Chaplinsky,R.J., Flier,J.S., Hunt,C.R., and Spiegelman,B.M. (1987). *Science,* **237,** 402.
10. Würzner,R., Morgan,H., Joysey,V., and Lachmann,P.J. (1993). *Molec. Immunol.*, **30,** 63.
11. Rooney,I.A., Atkinson,J.P., Krul,E.S., Schonfeld,G., Polakoski,K., Saffitz,J.E., and Morgan,B.P. (1993). *J. Exp. Med.*, **177,** 1409.
12. Lachmann,P.J. and Walport,M.J. (1987). In *Autoimmunity and autoimmune disease* (ed. J.Whelan,) p. 149. Ciba Foundation Symposium, Vol. **129.** Wiley, Chichester.
13. Schifferli,J.A., Woo,P., and Peters,D.K. (1982). *Clin. Exp. Immunol.*, **47,** 555.
14. Miller,G.W. and Nussenzweig,V. (1975). *Proc. Natl Acad. Sci. USA,* **72,** 418.
15. Davies,K.A., Hird,V., Stewart,S., Sivolapenko,G.B., Jose,P., Epenetos,A.A., and Walport,M.J. (1990). *J. Immunol.*, **144,** 4613.
16. Davies,K.A., Erlendsson,K., Beynon,H.L., Peters,A.M., Steinsson,K., Valdimarsson,H., and Walport,M.J. (1993). *J. Immunol.*, **151,** 3866.
17. Cornacoff,J.B., Hebert,L.A., Smead,W.L., VanAman,M.E., Birmingham,D.J., and Waxman,F.J. (1983). *J. Clin. Invest.*, **71,** 236.
18. Waxman,F.J., Hebert,L.A., Cornacoff,J.B., VanAman,M.E., Smead,W.L., Kraut,E.H., Birmingham,D.J., and Taguiam,J.M. (1984). *J. Clin. Invest.*, **74,** 1329.
19. Miller,G.W., Steinberg,A.D., Green,I., and Nussenzweig,V. (1975). *J. Immunol.*, **114,** 1166.

20. Fielder,A.H.L., Walport,M.J., Batchelor,J.R., Rynes,R.I., Black,C.M., Dodi,I.A., and Hughes,G.R.V. (1983). *Brit. Med. J. Clin. Res.*, **286**, 425.
21. Law,S.K.A., Dodds,A.W., and Porter,R.R. (1984). *EMBO J.*, **3**, 1819.
22. Gatenby,P.A., Barbosa,J.E., and Lachmann,P.J. (1990). *Clin. Exp. Immunol.*, **79**, 158.
23. Daha,M.R. (1987) In *Complement in health and disease* (ed. K.Whaley), p. 185. MTP, Lancaster.
24. Gorski,J., Hugli,T.E., and Müller-Eberhard,H.J. (1979). *Proc. Natl Acad. Sci. USA*, **76**, 5299.
25. Cochrane,C.G. and Müller-Eberhard,H.J. (1968). *J. Exp. Med.*, **127**, 371.
26. Marceau,F., Lundberg,C., and Hugli,T.E. (1987). *Immunopharmacology*, **14**, 67.
27. Fernandez,H.N., Henson,P.M., Otani,A., and Hugli,T.E. (1978). *J. Immunol.*, **120**, 109.
28. Miller,L.J., Bainton,D.F., Borregaard, N., and Springer,T.A. (1987). *J. Clin. Invest.*, **80**, 535.
29. Goldstein,I.M. and Weissmann,G. (1974). *J. Immunol.*, **113**, 1583.
30. Kurimoto,Y., de Weck,A.L., and Dahinden,C.A. (1989). *J. Exp. Med.*, **170**, 467.
31. Goldstein,I.M., Ross,D., Kaplan,H.B., and Weissmann,G. (1975). *J. Clin. Invest.*, **56**, 1155.
32. Wright,S.D. and Silverstein,S.C. (1982). *J. Exp. Med.*, **156**, 1149.
33. Wright,S.D. and Silverstein,S.C. (1983). *J. Exp. Med.*, **158**, 2016.
34. Wright,S.D., Craigmyle,L.S., and Silverstein,S.C. (1983). *J. Exp. Med.*, **158**, 1338.
35. Newman,S.L., Mikus,L.K., and Tucci,M.A. (1991). *J. Immunol.*, **146**, 967.
36. Brown,E.J., Bohnsack,J.F., and Gresham,H.D. (1988). *J. Clin. Invest.*, **8**, 365.
37. Graham,I.L., Gresham,H.D., and Brown,E.J. (1989). *J. Immunol.*, **142**, 2352.
38. Axline,S.G. and Reaven,E.P. (1974). *J. Cell Biol.*, **62**, 647.
39. Bobak,D.A., Gaither,T.A., Frank,M.M., and Tenner,A.J. (1987). *J. Immunl.*, **38**, 1150.
40. Guan,E., Burgess,W.H., Robinson,S.L., Goodman,E.B., McTigue,K.J., and Tenner,A.J. (1991). *J. Biol. Chem.*, **266**, 20345.
41. Hamada,A., Young,J., Chmielewski,R.A., and Greene,B.M. (1988). *J. Clin. Invest.*, **82**, 945.
42. Podack,E.R. (1986). In *Immunobiology of the complement system* (ed. G.D.Ross), p. 115. Academic Press, London.
43. Ohanian,S.H. and Schlager,S.I. (1981). *CRC Crit. Rev. Immunol.*, **1**, 165.
44. Joiner,K., Brown,E., Hammer,C., Warren,K., and Frank,M. (1983). *J. Immunol.*, **130**, 845.
45. Clas,F. and Loos,M. (1987). In *Complement in health and disease* (ed. K.Whaley), p. 201. MTP, Lancaster.
46. Ogata,R.T. and Levine,R.P. (1980). *J. Immunol.*, **125**, 1494.
47. Ruppel,A. (1987). In *Complement in health and disease* (ed. K.Whaley), p. 233. MTP Press, Lancaster.
48. Sissons,J.G.P. (1987). In *Complement in health and disease* (ed. K.Whaley), p. 255. MTP, Lancaster.
49. Ahearn,J.M. and Fearon,D.T. (1989). *Adv. Immunol.*, **46**, 183.
50. Dorig,R.E., Marcil,A., Chopra,A., and Richardson,C.D. (1993). *Cell*, **75**, 295.
51. Naniche,D., Varior-Krishnan,G., Cervoni,F., Wild,T.F., Rossi,B., Rabourdin-Combe,C., and Gerlier,D. (1993). *J. Virol.*, **67**, 6025.
52. Dierich,M.P., Ebenbichler,C.F., Marschang,P., Füst,G., Thielens,N.M., and Arlaud,G.J. (1993). *Immunol. Today*, **14**, 435.
53. Boyer,V., Dilibrias,C., Noraz,N., Fischer,E., Kazatchkine,M.D., and Desgranges,C. (1992). *Scand. J. Immunol.*, **36**, 879.

54. Reisinger,E.C., Vogetseder,W., Berzow,D., Kofler,D., Bitterlich,G., Lehr,H.A., Wachter,H., and Dierich,M.P. (1990). *AIDS*, **4,** 961.
55. Böttger,E.C., Hoffmann,T., Hadding,U., and Bitter-Suermann,D. (1985). *J. Immunol.*, **135,** 4100.
56. Finco,O., Li,S., Cuccia,M., Rosen,F.S., and Carroll,M.C. (1992). *J. Exp. Med.*, **175,** 537.
57. Pepys,M.B. (1976). *Transpl. Rev.*, **32,** 93.
58. Feldman,M. and Pepys,M.B. (1974). *Nature*, **249,** 159.
59. Meuth,J.L., Morgan,E.L., DiScipio,R.G., and Hugli,T.E. (1983). *J. Immunol.*, **130,** 2605.
60. Melchers,F., Erdei,A., Schulz,T., and Dierich,M.P. (1985). *Nature*, **317,** 264.
61. Heyman,B., Wiersma,E.J., and Kinoshita,T. (1990). *J. Exp. Med.*, **172,** 665.
62. Hebell,T., Ahearn,J.M., and Fearon,D.T. (1991). *Science*, **254,** 102.
63. Fearon,D.T. (1993) *Clin. Opin. Immunol.*, **5,** 341.
64. Carter,R.H. and Fearon,D.T. (1992). *Science*, **258,** 105.
65. Haicht,G.S., Beck,G., and Ghebrehiwet,B. (1987). *J. Immunol.*, **138,** 2593.
66. Köhl,J. and Bitter-Suermann,D. (1993). In *Complement in health and disease* (ed. K.Whaley, M.Loos, and J.M.Weiler), p. 299. Immunology and Medicine Series 20. Kluwer Academic, London.
67. Masden,H.O., Garred,P., Kurtzhals,J.A.L., Lamm,L.U., Ryder,L.P., Thiel,S., and Svejgaard,A. (1994). *Immunogenetics*, **40,** 37.
68. Super,M., Thiel,S., Lu,J., Levinsky,R.J., and Turner,M.W. (1989). *Lancet*, **2,** 1236.
69. Tosi,M. (1993). In *Complement in health and disease* (ed. K.Whaley, M.Loos, and J.M.Weiler), p. 245. Immunology and Medicine Series **20.** Kluwer Academic, London.
70. Bessler,M., Mason,P.J., Hillmen,P., Miyata,T., Yamada,N., Takeda,J., Luzzatto, L., and Kinoshita,T. (1994). *EMBO J.*, **13,** 110.
71. Yamashina,M., Udea,E., Kinoshita,T., Takami,T., Ojima,A., Ono,H., Tanaka,H., Kondo,N., Orii,T., Okada,N., Okada,H., Inoue,K., and Kitani,T. (1990). *New Engl. J. Med.*, **323,** 1184.
72. Arnaout,M.A. (1990). *Immunol. Rev.*, **114,** 145.
73. Janatova,J., Cheung,A.K., and Parker,C.J. (1990). *Complement Inflamm.*, **8,** 61.
74. Weisman,H.F., Bartow,T., Leppo,M.K., Marsh,H.C.J., Carson,G.R., Concino,M.F., Boyle,M.P., Roux,K.H., Weisfeldt,M.L., and Fearon,D.T. (1990). *Science*, **249,** 146.
75. Arfors,K.E., Lundberg,C., Lindbom,L., Lundberg,K., Beatty,P.G., and Harlan,J.M. (1987). *Blood*, **69,** 338.
76. Rosen,H. and Gordon,S. (1987). *J. Exp. Med.*, **166,** 1685.
77. Sakiyalak,P., Leventhal, J.R., Witson,J., Bolman,R.M., and Dalmasso,A.P. (1993). *Mol. Immunol.*, **30,** 49.
78. Xia,W., Fearon,D.T., Moore,F.D., Jr., Schoen,F.J., Ortiz,F., and Kirkman,R.L. (1992). *Transplant. Proc.*, **24,** 479.
79. Miyagawa,S., Shirakura,R., Matsuda,H., Iwata,K., Matsumoto,M., Seya,T., and Nagasawa,S. (1993). *Mol. Immunol.*, **30,** 33.
80. Whaley,K. (1987). In *Complement in health and disease* (ed. K. Whaley), p. 163. MTP, Lancaster.
81. Schreiber,R.D., Morrison,D.C., Podack,E.R., and Müller-Eberhard,H.J. (1979). *J. Exp. Med.*, **149,** 870.
82. Schifferli,J.A. and Peters,D.K. (1983). *Lancet*, **2,** 957.

Glossary

Activation of complement: the process by which enzymatically active complement fragments and the membrane attack complex are generated.

Alternative pathway/amplification loop: a pathway which results in C3 activation involving factors B, D, P, and C3b, and the control protein factors H and I. Activation is triggered in the presence of activator molecules and surfaces such as components of bacterial and fungal cell walls. In the presence of activators the pathway activation is self-reinforcing and therefore acts to amplify the initial C3 activation, hence it is referred to as an amplification loop.

Anaphylatoxins: the fragments C3a, C4a, and C5a which, by their actions on the vasculature and smooth muscle, produce symptoms of anaphylaxis.

Chemotaxis: the directional movement of cells up a concentration gradient of a chemotactic molecule, for example C5a.

Classical pathway: a pathway which results in C3 activation, involving C1, C4, and C2, which is triggered usually by the binding of C1q to antigen–antibody complexes.

Complement receptors: membrane proteins which, by binding with various complement activation fragments, trigger the appropriate cellular responses.

Convertases: molecular complexes which can enzymatically cleave particular components (for example, C3-convertases split C3 into C3a and C3b).

Decay acceleration: the C3- and C5-convertases decay naturally by the dissociation of the catalytic components, namely factor Bb or C2a, from the cofactor components, which are C3b and C4b. This dissociation may be accelerated by some members of the RAC proteins including factor H, C4bp, DAF, and CR1.

Enzyme cascade: a description of several plasma enzyme systems, including complement, in which the activation of one component generates an enzyme which acts on the next component in the activation sequence thus each step is an amplification of the previous one.

Lectin route of activation: activation of complement initiated by mannan binding protein (MBP), which, via its lectin modules, binds to carbohydrate structures found on bacteria and other microorganisms. A MBP-associated serine protease (MASP) becomes activated and it, in turn, can split and activate the complement components C4 and C2. MBP is analogous to C1q and MASP to C1r and C1s.

Membrane attack complex (MAC): a molecular complex formed by C5b, C6, C7, C8, and a number of C9 molecules which can integrate into plasma membrane and cause cell lysis.

MHC class III genes: the region of the major histocompatibility complex between the regions containing genes for the class I and class II antigens. The complement genes for C2, factor B, and the two C4 isotypes C4A and C4B are four of the many (35 to date) genes characterized in this region.

Opsonization: the process by which antigenic material becomes coated with molecules (e.g. IgG and C3b) which facilitate their uptake by phagocytes.

Perforin: protein which is secreted by cytotoxic T cells and which is involved in causing lysis of target cells.

Phagocytosis: the ingestion of opsonized targets by macrophages or neutrophils after initial adhesion of the phagocytes to the targets via FcR-IgG, CR1-C3b, and CR3-iC3b interactions.

Pro-enzyme: an enzymatically inactive molecule which may become enzymatically active by proteolytic cleavage.

Regulators of complement activation (RCA): the group of proteins including factors H, C4bp, DAF, MCP, CR1, and CR2 whose genes are located in a cluster on chromosome 1q32. These proteins are composed predominantly of CCP repeats, and they all interact with the C3 and C4 activated fragments.

Terminal pathway (lytic pathway): the pathway involving C5 to C9 which generates the membrane attack complex.

Thiolester: the chemical structure –S–CO–. In the case of the complement proteins C3 and C4, the bond is formed between a –SH group on a cysteine residue and a $-CONH_2$ group on a glutamine residue with the elimination of NH_3. The cysteine and the glutamine residues are in the tetrapeptide sequence –Cys –Gly–Glu–Gln–. Activation of the C3 and C4 allows their activated fragments, C3b and C4b, to bind covalently to target cell surfaces via the acyl group of the Gln residue.

Index